Temporomandibular Disorders

Temporomandibular Disorders

William K. Solberg, DDS, MDS

Professor and Chair, Section of Gnathology and Occlusion,
Director, Temporomandibular and Facial Pain Clinic,
School of Dentistry, Center for Health Sciences,
University of California, Los Angeles,
California USA

1986

Published by the British Dental Association
64 Wimpole Street, London W1M 8AL

Papers reprinted from the
British Dental Journal
March 8 to June 21, 1986

British Library Cataloguing in Publication Data
Solberg William K
Temporomandibular Disorders
1. Temporomandibular joint—Diseases
I. Title
617'522 RK470
ISBN 0 904588 16 5

Printed in England by
E T Heron (Print) Ltd, Silver End,
Witham, Essex

Acknowledgements

I am grateful to Margaret Seward, Editor of the *British Dental Journal*, for offering me the opportunity to write a series of papers on temporomandibular disorders. Michael Wise and Assistant Editor, Helen Goodier are especially thanked for their research and editorial contributions. I am indebted to Irene Petravicius of Dental Illustration and Richard Friske of Dental Photography at the School of Dentistry, University of California, for their contributions. I acknowledge the productive discussions and stimulating working relationships with my colleagues, Carole-Ann Bibb, Glen T. Clerk and Andrew G. Pullinger. Lastly, I would like to express my gratitude to my wife, Patricia Smiley, whose encouragement was most helpful.

Foreword

The *BDJ* Teach-In is an eagerly awaited regular fixture in the Postgraduate Dental Calendar. Since its inception in 1979, the invited lecturers have covered a wide spectrum of subjects encompassing clinical dentistry as well as practice management topics. However, the choice of the temporomandibular joint for the 1986 Teach In is a topic guaranteed to provoke discussion and controversy among dentists worldwide. Although the last twenty-five years has produced a vast number of articles written about investigation, treatment and management of the TMJ, the Journal has only occasionally published an article as a contribution to the debate. Therefore, I have invited Dr William Solberg, who has previously lectured on this topic in the USA, to write a series of articles for the Journal. Dr Solberg is the Director of Temporomandibular and Facial Pain Clinic, and a member of the Dental Research Institute at the University of California, Los Angeles. He is also Professor and Chairman of the Section of Gnathology and Occlusion at the Dental School.

This book is published to accompany the seventh Teach In and is an important addition to the rapidly growing list of titles published by the *British Dental Journal*.

Margaret Seward
Editor
September 1986

Preface

Functional disorders and facial pain in the temporomandibular region are common problems facing the dentist, even though the pathophysiological basis for their treatment is only now being realised. Clear understanding of this problem has not been achieved in dentistry because the knowledge base is scattered over many areas such as physiology, orthopaedics, rheumatology, psychology, and neurology. Nevertheless, the management of temporomandibular disorders by the dentist is justified both on anatomical grounds and by the positive results of good treatment outcomes achieved using practical measures in the dental surgery. Gaining a better perspective on the diagnosis and management of temporomandibular disorders by the dentist is the aim of this book.

Contents

1 Background and the clinical problems

The purpose of this book is to provide an approach to problems of temporomandibular (TM) disorders in the dental practice setting. This series is also presented in response to the often stated desire among practitioners to gain more competence in this rapidly growing area of dental practice. A recent poll[1] of 5000 dentists in the USA revealed a significant increase in aesthetic dentistry, preventive dentistry, and TMJ therapy. There was a concomitant decrease in paedodontics, complete dentures, and oral surgery.

The difficulty surrounding the management of patients with TM disorders is evident. Some of these problems reflect dentists' rigid perceptions of their role, a real lack of scientific information, and a lack of training on the nature and management of TM disorders. Surrounding these issues is the dentists' uneasiness in coping with psychosocial factors associated with multifactorial disease. A factor generating great inertia in the field is the status of professional reimbursement for TM disorder procedures in the health care system. This factor is not within the scope of this paper but is mentioned for consideration by the reader elsewhere.[2]

Gaining a better perspective on the problem of TM disorders is the aim of this introductory article. We will delve into various problem compartments which, despite much recent progress, are incomplete or lacking practical resolution at this time.

Dentists' rituals in practice
Dentists have a historic role in resolving acute pain and in restoring oral

function. We have been taught to seek specific structural explanations for pain and for malfunction. Furthermore, dental training has traditionally emphasised technical skill in manipulating tools and materials and in fashioning prosthetic devices. A carious molar, a missing incisor, an infected peridontium, a crowded arch: these are the problems that dentists routinely and quickly evaluate and then competently solve.

When confronted with patients who appear suffering from obscure facial pain and functional jaw problems, dentists are forced to adjust their habitual focus. They are less quick and less comfortable when confronted with clicking joints, sore muscles, limited mouth openings, and other obscure disorders that may not always suggest specific treatment. Managing these patients and their problems requires the dentist to change his emphasis from the tangibles of treatment planning to the uncertainties of medical diagnosis.

The shift in emphasis might be described as follows: dentists have customarily provided a product or a procedure; in this instance they will be called upon to provide a primary care service. Although dentists are broadening their skills and mix of services they provide, never has this expanded role been better exemplified than by the dentist's involvement in treating TM disorders. It is particularly important that dentists should treat TM pain and dysfunction, since their special knowledge can be employed with material effect in treatment of these disorders.

Despite these clear obligations, the path to competence in this area is not straightforward. The lack of dental training and research in this area has left dentists sorely confused. The confusion has created a polarisation whereby one school of thought believes the problem to be psychological or functional, while others believe these problems to be mechanical or occlusal in origin. Between those two groups are the largest group of professionals: those who are wholly indifferent. Dentists' indifference to obscure facial pain is not only traumatic to sufferers but also to dentists, leading to untold patient dissatisfaction with practitioners and frustration with their neglect. A fair amount of iatrogenic adventurism is concomitantly invited as dentists are pressed to work on the fringes of their abilities.

Temporomandibular disorders as recognisable ailments

Temporomandibular disorders are musculoskeletal problems surfacing in a non-traditional area, the head and jaws. Professionals who normally see patients with head and face pain or jaw dysfunction have little background in the management of problems emanating from muscles and synovial joints. The surgical model of acute pain and disease, findings which dentists have used with great success, has not been successful when applied to acquired benign pain. It is not surprising, therefore, that the field is characterised by diverse approaches in management with inevitable controversy and incompetence.

A more appropriate diagnostic framework is needed better to characterise TM disorders as recognisable ailments. The framework is found in the domain of acquired connective tissue disorders, collectively termed soft tissue musculoskeletal or neuromuscular pain and dysfunction. The site of the problem, the soft tissues, is not considered an organ system and therefore is poorly defined and not well taught in professional training.[3] The temporomandibular joint is unquestionably difficult to observe, and therefore the anatomical site has been understudied by clinicians. For the most part, dentists have neglected the TMJ in favour of more obvious problems of the teeth and the oral cavity. Orthodontists have focused on craniofacial growth and development with concomitant neglect of the implications of craniofacial orthopaedics. It is now important for dentists to develop their treatment concepts using methodologies proven for the management of other synovial joints and myofascial systems.

Scope and cause
Definition
Attempts to assess the scope of TM disorders begin with a definition of the problem. Temporomandibular disorders are musculoskeletal discomfort or dysfunction in the masticatory system aggravated by chewing or other jaw use but independent of local disease involving the teeth and mouth. Pain in the masticatory system independent of oral function, such as pulpitis or cervical strain causing referred masticatory pain, is not a TM disorder.[4] The diagnosis of a TM disorder should be made after appropriate criteria (Table I). TM disorders should not be used as a catch-all term for any facial pain.

The signature of the TM disorder is pain provoked by function. Pain and dysfunction go hand in hand. Resting pain unrelated to jaw function is much less common and should direct the clinician to suspect alternative disorders.[4] We are not identifying one illness, however, that has clearly identifiable features. We must be able to identify subtypes of TM disorders in order to render an appropriate treatment plan and prognosis (Table II). In addition, these conditions have unique and complex aetiologies and may affect various sites of the masticatory system. For example, TM disorders can manifest themselves as disc derangements in the TMJ following a direct blow, troublesome jaw and head pain related to nocturnal bruxism, and acute muscle spasm following prolonged jaw extension at the dentist.

The general term for these musculoskeletal conditions, temporomandibular disorder, has been adopted by the American Dental Association in their publications.[5]

Symptoms

The symptoms of TM disorders are well known and generally agreed upon.[6] Functional jaw pain, TMJ incoordination and restriction of jaw movement make up the classic triad against a background of lesser and more varied symptoms. However, on the basis of recent studies[7-9] recurrent headache must be elevated to the list of major symptoms. The difficulty in separating TM disorder headaches from muscle contraction headaches[9] and their amelioration by TMJ treatment[10] now justify this approach. Pincus and Tucker[11] stated that headaches caused by TM disorder were more common in their neurological practice than migraine headaches (26% and 20% respectively). In addition, Gregg[12] pointed out the intriguing possibility that masticatory myfascial pain may have a vascular component. Naturally, since the term headache covers a vast field of identifiable conditions, the treatment of headaches from the masticatory viewpoint should be discouraged in the absence of other TM disorder symptoms.

Epidemiology

Over twenty epidemiological investigations have been performed on non-patient populations since the 1970s. (For a review of these studies see Rugh and Solberg.[13]) The basic message is that the clinician can anticipate finding one patient in four who is aware of symptoms, while almost two in four display clinical abnormalities qualitatively similar to those found in patients with TM complaints. The features that distinguish patients reporting for treatment are mainly relative ones: frequency, persistence,

Table I Identification and localisation of temporomandibular disorders (after Bell)[3]

Temporomandibular pain
(1) The pain should relate directly and logically to movements and function incidental to mastication
(2) Tenderness in the masticatory muscles or over the TMJs should be obvious from manual palpation
(3) Analgesic blocking of the tender muscle or the joint should confirm the presence and location of the pain source

Temporomandibular dysfunction
(1) Interference with mandibular movement (clicking, incoordination, crepitus)
(2) Restriction of mandibular movement (limitation of normal movement patterns)
(3) Sudden changes in the occlusal relationships of the teeth

---

Table II Clinical classification of TM disorders

Acute masticatory muscle disorders
TMJ derangement (includes hypermobility)
TMJ inflammatory disorders
Degenerative disease (non-inflammatory)
Extrinsic trauma
Chronic hypomobility
Growth disorders

and severity of symptoms. The clinician is therefore cautioned not to classify individuals who demonstrate these symptoms as clinically ill. Obviously, recommending treatment after merely detecting symptoms and signs is clinical overkill.

For approximately 5% of individuals, however, the condition represents a significant problem at some period in their lives.[13] Most people who encounter painful dysfunction will experience it before the age of 40 years. Some patients, most above 40 years, suffer from osteoarthritis which is a late stage of the TM disorder.[14] It should be noted that Ogus[15] has described some forms of TMJ degenerative disease in young persons. Women predominate among patient groups in a ratio of greater than 3:1. Therefore, the target group for therapy appears to be women between the ages of 15 and 40 years.

Symptom progression
Temporomandibular disorders have their own natural history. They form a continuum of subclinical symptoms that are often self-limiting, adaptive states. Indeed, many patients who have severe TMJ radiographic changes have never had that joint become symptomatic. With disease progression and increasing severity of symptoms, however, the problem becomes one of personal significance to the individual causing them to seek treatment (fig. 1). Treatment is not the same for all stages on the progression. Thus, pattern recognition is important in patient evaluation.

Aetiology
Understanding the aetiology of TM disorders is not straightforward. Both central and peripheral factors appear to be important with both morphofunctional (occlusion, bruxism) and psychological factors (anxiety, tension) implicated as multifactorial causes.[16] The clinical significance of this approach is to call attention to the necessity for dealing with the aetiological factors as well as the symptoms in diagnosis and in treatment (fig. 2).

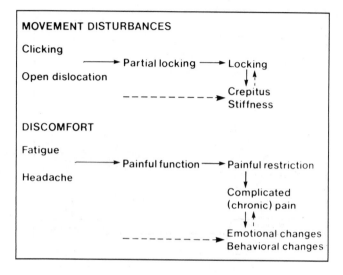

Fig. 1 Progression of temporomandibular disorders (from Solberg W K. Current concepts on the development of TMJ dysfunction. *In* Carlson D, McNamara J A Jr and Ribbens K A (eds) *Developmental aspects of temporomandibular disorders*, pp 37–47. Ann Arbor: University of Michigan, 1985).

Recently Pullinger *et al.*[17] showed that the factor of trauma was significantly associated with symptoms when this historical factor was studied in a TMJ patient and comparison group. Brook and Sten[18] showed that a less favourable outcome is associated with post-injury TM disorders. In view of these findings, trauma appears to be important as a causal factor.

Long term impact of temporomandibular disorders
Life history
Consideration of the history of a disease may be a novel idea to many dentists accustomed to identifying an immediate problem, such as caries, and treating it in a definitive way. With temporomandibular disorders, however, a less aggressive role is warranted. Pain and dysfunction should be considered in light of their chronicity and progression (fig. 1); treatment is instituted when the natural course of symptoms appears to warrant therapeutic support.

The expected clinical course of TM disorders ranges widely from 10 days to five years. Often these disorders are recurrent or even constant over a greater period of time. Rasmussen, in a six-year longitudinal patient study,[19] documented that 'TMJ arthropathy' consisted of three stages:

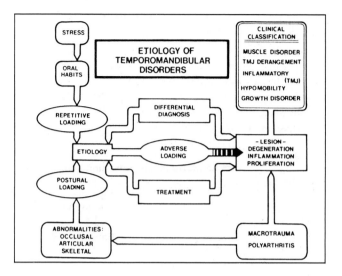

Fig. 2 Aetiological pathways of temporomandibular disorders according to the multifactorial concept. Temporomandibular disorders result from adverse loading of the jaw system, differentially generated by repetitive loadings due to stress, postural loading due to biomechanical factors, and macrotrauma (from Solberg W K, Seligman D A. Temporomandibular orthopedics: A new vista in orthodontics. *In* Johnston L E (ed) *New Vistas in Orthodontics,* pp 148-183. Philadelphia:Lea and Febiger, 1985).

(1) initial stage—clicking and locking,

(2) intermediate stage—TMJ pain and restriction,

(3) terminal stage—crepitation and constriction, often followed by symptom resolution.

The three stages were found to have a duration of four years, one year, and half a year respectively. Complete recovery was most favourable for those with intact dentitions or complete dentures, indicating that the rate of healing from TMJ arthropathy may depend to some degree on dental status.[19] Overall, much more information on the natural course of TM disorders is needed. The situation is complicated by the fact that these disorders fluctuate over time and may dissipate with or without treatment.

Need for treatment

It is not clear at this time which signs and symptoms of TM disorders should signal the need for intervention by the clinician. At present, it is not established how many individuals with early signs and symptoms develop serious conditions.[13] The dysfunctional index reviewed by Helkimo[20] has helped establish guidelines for need of treatment, but it has limitations in characterising the exact clinical state of the TMJ patient.

Considering TM disorders in their larger domain, there is evidence that muscle and joint pains, especially those in the upper quarter of the body, are a major cause of workdays lost[21] (fig. 3). Visits for headache, in particular, are in part due to head pain secondary to TM disorders.[8] Not enough is known about the natural history of the various TM disorder conditions to make clear what preventive procedures should be taken. As more is understood about the various conditions, there may be a considerable need for preventive measures.[13]

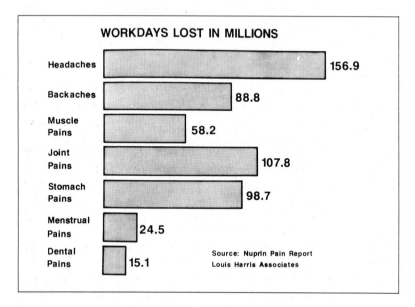

Fig. 3 Workdays lost in millions (from Harris L and Associates. The Nuprin pain report. Study no. 851017. New York: Louis Harris and Associates Inc., 1985).

Table III Deep somatic and visceral pain characteristics (after Bell[3])

Depressive
Dull quality
Poorly localisable
Source may be remote
Secondary central excitatory effects
    Referred pain
    Secondary hyperalgesia
    Localised autonomic symptoms
    Skeletal muscle effects

Demand for treatment

Of the total population from western countries, the percentage of individuals who seek treatment for TM disorders ranges from 3 to 7%.[13] All observers agree that the demand is increasing, mostly related to offers of care by dentists, to increased trauma from vehicular accidents, and to increased awareness of lay persons. In short, there probably has been a real increase in the incidence of TM disorders but the evidence is sparse. It is not clear at this time what increases may relate to overtreatment by dentists who believe that even minor signs or symptoms should be treated. There clearly is no evidence to support mandatory treatment for all symptoms.[13] Thus, dentists have been encouraged by the American Dental Association's presidential task force on TMJ to use palliative, reversible therapy.[5]

Disability

TM disorders are not life threatening; their treatment relates to improvement in the quality of life. Faulty or painful function disturbs eating, sexual activity, sleep, speech, non-verbal communication, and body image. These disabilities, arising from deep, ineffable sources, become so significant as to impair an individual's emotional stability. Some individuals are seriously troubled by perceived alterations in the character of their mouth and jaws. They develop a great sense of deformity, which can be exacerbated by dentists' and physicians' dismissing the problem as illegitimate because it is not demonstrable on radiograph or by visual examination.

Temporomandibular disorders produce the attributes of deep pain, including secondary central excitatory[22] effects (Table III). This is more likely to happen if the pain is constant as well as severe. Therefore, a worthy goal in TMJ therapy is to take steps to control constant pain.[22] When central excitatory effects are present, TM disorders can be confusing and mysterious to the clinician naive about the general attributes of deep somatic and visceral pain.

When TMJ dysfunction induces chronic pain, the patient's threshold for pain is altered. The pain experience can cause patients to learn to be invalids, profiting from secondary gain through attention, substitution for aggression, and expression of grief.[6] A debilitating cycle is established that reinforces pain (fig. 1).

Accepted treatments

Referred pain and variety of regional complaints such as unilateral earaches, neckaches, headaches plus dizziness, ear stuffiness and ringing of

Table IV Potential procedures for temporomandibular disorders

Explanation and counselling	Mobilisation and manipulation incorporating vapocoolant spray and anaesthetic blockade
Temporomandibular joint radiograms (orthopantomograms, transcranials, tomograms, arthrograms)	Diathermy and moist heat
Stress management, biofeedback	Transdermal stimulation and acupuncture
Pharmacotherapy	Bite appliances and occlusal adjustment of the teeth
Therapeutic exercises	Arthroscopic therapy and arthroplasty

Table V—Symptoms before and after treatment in 151 patients with temporomandibular disorders (%). (From Majersjö C, Carlsson G E. Long term results of treatment for temporomandibular pain and dysfunction. *J Prosthet Dent* 1983; **49**: 809–815.)

	Before	Interim	7-year follow-up
TMJ noise	56	42	23
Tiredness and stiffness	29	44	12
Limited oral opening	35	13	7
Pain on mandibular movement	39	10	5
Facial pain (excluding dental pain and headache)	69	22	8
Locking and/or dislocation	20	11	0

the ears cause patients to see a wide variety of doctors. This action has spawned an impressive number of treatments, some appropriate, others without basis. Fortunately, with more productive inquiry by clinicians and researchers, a treatment matrix is emerging and gaining general acceptance (Table IV). Since temporomandibular joint pain and dysfunction is a musculoskeletal problem, it is treated with the same therapies appropriate for other joints and muscles, namely:

(1) rest;

(2) physical therapy;

(3) bite appliances for stabilisation of the temporomandibular joints and dental occlusion.

Emotional factors (such as anxiety, fear, frustration, and anger) play a role in the aetiology of TM disorders; behaviour modification and stress management are often helpful. Dental procedures are often utilised in the form of orthopaedic appliances and bite adjustment for stabilising the muscle and joint structures. Moreover, patients are directed to their general dentist for permanent treatment to the teeth when necessary. If structural derangements occur in the soft or hard tissues of the joint, and if more conservative measures prove ineffective, surgical intervention may be warranted.

Outcome of treatment

The average duration of treatment for patients is approximately three months, with appointments scheduled every two or three weeks. Approximately 80% of patients with this disorder have good to excellent relief with conservative treatment procedures.

Despite the common use of many modalities in treating TM disorders, few longitudinal outcome studies have been conducted. The enormous difficulty encountered in conducting such studies has outweighed their acknowledged value in providing information vital to proper decision making. A major scientific roadblock in conducting these studies has been the lack of definitive criteria for identifying the TMJ case.[23] It is noteworthy that TM disorders are among many soft tissue disorders, headaches, neckaches, and backache, that are lacking adequate outcome studies.

In a seven-year follow-up study, Majersjö and Carlsson[24] reported that most patients are considerably better, particularly if they have undergone rather uncomplicated forms of dental treatment and self-care regimens (Table V).

In a retrospective review of 350 patients, Wedell and Carlsson[25] found the average visits to number four and the average duration of treatment to be three months. Although the extent of treatment was widely variable, the initial severity of signs and symptoms, especially muscle tenderness, was associated with length of treatment. Initial severity, however, could not be found to bear on the patients' status at follow-up $2\frac{1}{2}$ years later. Dental occlusion factors were not well correlated to treatment outcome, except that dentate individuals were more apt to undergo lengthy treatments. On the basis of these initial studies, a good prognosis can be conveyed to patients noting that they can be helped by the effects of rather simple treatment.[25]

Conclusion

The temporomandibular joint and associated myoligamentous structures are subject to wear and tear and injury not unlike other synovial joints. Because articular tissues are tough and avascular, they may not heal properly when injured. Because TM disorders cause chronic pain, the patient becomes anxious and depressed and shows signs of anxiety.

Patients with TM disorders present a challenge to the dentist because their condition represents a curious combination of psychological and somatic manifestations. It is notable that both the obscurity of the problem and the lack of adequate orientation on the part of the dentist confound its management. Nevertheless, the diagnosis of TM disorders can be suspected on the basis of specific criteria, and it is more firmly established when other observable causes of regional pain and dysfunction have been excluded. Because subliminal symptoms are plentiful in otherwise healthy individuals, controversy continues as to what represents functional adaptation in contrast to pathologic lesions.

The fundamental unanswered question is what causes these disorders, and why they are disproportionately bothersome in younger adult women. There may be a key mechanism that dominates all others, but it will take a long time to elucidate. Meanwhile, the development of reliable principles of diagnosis and management is a continuing challenge which this series of eight papers intends to address.

References

1   Clinical Research Associates Newsletter. 1–4pp. 9 (10): Provo: Utah, USA 1985.
2   Prepayment plan benefits for temporomandibular joint disorders. Council on Dental Care Programs. *J Am Dent Assoc* 1982; **105**: 485-488.
3   Caillet R. *Soft tissue pain and disability.* Philadelphia: F. A. Davis Co, 1977.
4   Bell W E. *Clinical management of temporomandibular disorders.* Chicago: Yearbook Medical Publishers, 1982.
5   Laskin D, Greenfield W, Gale E. *et al. The president's conference on the examination, diagnosis, and management of temporomandibular disorders.* Chicago: The American Dental Association, 1982.
6   Rugh J D, Solberg W K. Psychological implications in temporomandibular joint function and dysfunction. *In* Zarb G, Carlsson G E (eds), *Temporomandibular joint function and dysfunction.* Copenhagen: Munksgaard, 1979.
7   Magnusson T, Carlsson G E. Recurrent headaches in relation to temporomandibular joint pain dysfunction. *Acta Odont Scand* 1978; **36**: 333-338.
8   Forssell H, Kangasniemi P. Correlation of the frequency and intensity of headache to mandibular dysfunction in headache patients. *Proc Finn Dent Soc* 1984; **80:** 223-226.
9   Reik Jr L, Hale M. The temporomandibular joint pain-dysfunction syndrome: A frequent cause of headache. *Headache* 1981; **21:** 51-156.
10 Magnusson T, Carlsson G E. Comparison between two groups of patients in respect of headache and mandibular dysfunction. *Swed Dent J* 1978; **2:** 85-92.
11 Pincus J H, Tucker G J. *Behavioral neurology.* 2nd ed. New York: Oxford University Press, 1978.
12 Gregg J M. Pharmacological management of myofascial pain dysfunction. *In:* Laskin D, Greenfield W, Gale E *et al.* (eds) *The president's conference on the examination, diagnosis, and management of temporomandibular disorders.* Chicago: The American Dental Association, 1983.

13 Rugh J D, Solberg W K. Oral health status in the United States: temporomandibular disorders. *J Dent Ed* 1985; **49:** 398–405.

14 Toller P A. Osteoarthrosis of the mandibular condyle. *Brit Dent J* 1973; **134:** 223–231.

15 Ogus H. Degenerative disease of the temporomandibular joint in young persons. *Brit J of Oral Surg* 1979–80; **17:** 17–26.

16 Solberg W K. Current concepts on the development of TMJ dysfunction. *In* Carlson D, McNamara J A Jr, Ribbens K A (eds.) *Developmental aspects of temporomandibular disorders*, pp 37–47. Ann Arbor: University of Michigan, 1985.

17 Pullinger A G, Montiero A, Lui S. Etiological factors associated with temporomandibular disorders. *J Dent Res* 1985; **64:** 269, abstract 848.

18 Brook R I, Sten P G. Postinjury myofascial pain dysfunction syndrome, its aetiology and prognosis. *J Oral Surg* 1978; **45:** 846–850.

19 Rasmussen O C. Description of population and progress of symptoms in a longitudinal study of temporomandibular arthropathy. *Scand J Dent Res* 1981; **89:** 196–203.

20 Helkimo M. Studies on function and dysfunction of the masticatory system. II. Index for anamnestic and clinical dysfunction and occlusal state. *Swed Dent J* 1974; **67:** 101–121.

21 Harris L and Associates. *The Nuprin pain report.* Study no. 851017. New York: Louis Harris and Associates Inc., 1985.

22 Bell W E. *Orofacial pains: classification diagnosis management.* 3rd ed, pp 61–72. Chicago: Year Book Medical Publishers Inc., 1985.

23 Katz R V. Response—oral health status in the United States: Temporomandibular disorders. *J Dent Ed* 1985; **49:** 406.

24 Majersjö C, Carlsson G E. Long term results of treatment for temporomandibular pain and dysfunction. *J Prosthet Dent* 1983; **49:** 809–815.

25 Wedel A, Carlsson G. Factors in influencing the outcome of treatment in patients referred to a temporomandibular joint clinic. *J Prosthet Dent* 1985; **54:** 420–426.

2 Functional and radiological considerations

The temporomandibular joint (TMJ), also known as the craniomandibular articulation,[1] is peculiar to mammals and has many distinctive characteristics. The articular zone of the TMJ differs from most synovial joints in that the articular surfaces consist of fibrous connective tissue, not hyaline cartilage. Factors of embryology and the need for the TMJs to withstand twisting, turning, compressive forces are the most common explanations for this structural difference. Each temporomandibular articulation consists of two articular units that provide for combined hinge and gliding action. The two articular units share a common component: the intact articular disc. When an intracapsular disc is present, the joint is termed complex.[2] The hinge feature (lower articular unit) allows passive manipulation to approximately 26 mm interincisal opening. The gliding feature (upper articular unit) allows maximum gape in the upright posture while at the same time bringing the jaw to the brink of dislocation. It is when undergoing combined hinge and gliding movements that most pain and dysfunction occur. Only rarely is pure hinge movement affected by TMJ dysfunction. If functional TMJ restriction occurs, the limitation of motion will usually start at 26 mm interincisal opening.

Because the right and left articulations are joined by the mandible, the movement of one articulation directly affects the other. Further, since the upper and lower jaw carry teeth, their shape and position will influence some TMJ movements.[1] Considering this unique feature, it is appropriate to consider the mandible a bone stabilised by three functionally linked articulations: the dentition and the two TMJs. Alteration in one of these functional links is manifested by adaptive changes in the others. Abrupt changes brought about through tooth loss or obtrusive dental restorations increase the risk that this accommodation will be accompanied by clinical discomfort and faulty TMJ function. Due to the distant ramifications of dental interventions, there is more interest among dentists about functional jaw orthopaedics in the provision of their services. Much of the controversy surrounding the mystery of TMJ dysfunction stems from a lack of knowledge of normal TMJ function and from technical and diagnostic flaws in the interpretation of its radiographic image.

The purpose of this paper is to describe the anatomical features of the TMJ that establish the foundation for analysing TMJ function in the clinical setting. Contemporaneous radiographic projections are discussed where they apply to employment in patient diagnosis.

TMJ features of clinical interest

One can draw erroneous conclusions looking at dry skulls and jawbones, for it is the soft tissues of the TMJs that are the entities of its crippling disorders. The primary components of the soft tissues are the articular cartilage, the fibrous capsule and disc, and the synovial mechanism. Alterations in these tissues are manifested by instability of the ligamentous attachments, constriction and stiffness of the capsule, and friction and adhesions of the articular surfaces. Accompanying generalised and localised inflammatory conditions make themselves known by tenderness and pain or pain on function.

Articular tissue

The condyle and temporal articular components consist of the spongy bone, compact bone, and the soft articular tissue (figs 1(*a*)–(*c*) and 2). The articulating surfaces consist of fibrous connective tissue, not hyaline cartilage, and the term, fibrocartilage only becomes meaningful with increasing age. This fibrous connective tissue is renewed independently of the subjacent proliferating zone of the condylar cap. Owing to its fibrous connective tissue composition, the term articular cartilage tends to be misleading for the TMJ. Therefore, the term articular tissue will be used to denote the soft tissues overlying the bony components.[3]

In the healthy young joint, the articulating surfaces are characterised by smooth, gently rounded contours. In the sagittal plane, both the articular eminence[4] and the condyle[5] resemble a parobola. It has been shown that deviation from symmetrical contour is usually the result of articular remodelling, not merely random variation.[6] The thickness of the articular

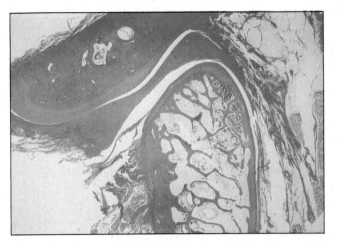

(a)

Fig. 1 Left TMJ taken at autopsy from an 18-year-old male with an intact dentition, embedded in celloidin and sectioned at 20-24 μm in a lateral plane at right angles to the horizontal condylar axis. (a) lateral third of the joint showing localised thickening in the articular tissue of the articular eminence and condyle

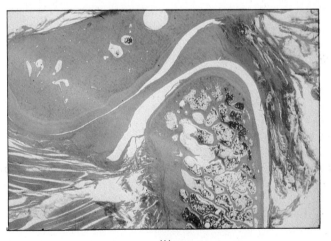

(b)

Middle third of the joint showing some localised thickening on the condyle

tissue normally varies from 0·1 to 0·5 mm, a relatively thin layer.[7] It is thickest on the superior aspect of the condyle and postero-inferior slope of the articular eminence. The articular tissue thickness may be even greater in areas of unusual functional loading. Figure 1(a) demonstrates localised

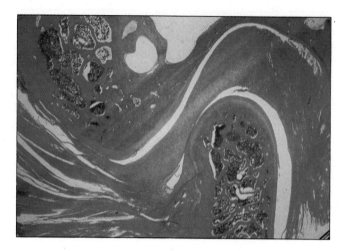

(c)
Medial third of the joint showing classic definition of the dense part of the disc and the bilaminar zone. Left side of figure is anterior. (From Solberg W K, and Hansson T L, Temporomandibular Joint Laboratory, UCLA Dental Research Institute, Los Angeles, California.)

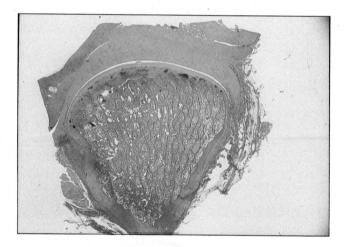

Fig. 2 Left TMJ taken at autopsy from a 21-year-old male with an intact dentition, embedded as in figure 1, and sectioned in a tilted frontal plane passing through the articular eminence and the condyle. Note the dense collagenous fibres of the medial discal attachment. The lateral discal attachment is not wholly in the plane of this section. Portions of the lateral ligament are observed to unite the temporal, discal and condylar components. Right side of figure is the lateral aspect. (Credits same as in figure 1.)

thickening on the postero-inferior slope of the articular eminence. Localised thickening can be seen on the superior aspect of the condyle in figure 1(*a*) and (*b*). The mandibular fossa is a dense but thin plate of compact bone covered by a thin soft tissue covering (periosteum). Obviously, this structure is not suited for functional loading (figs 1(*a*)–(*c*).

The articular disc is a meshwork of firmly woven avascular fibrous tissue. Its histological structure is therefore identical to the most superficial tissue layer covering the condylar and temporal articular surfaces. The healthy articular disc is thin at its centre with a functionally important thick anterior band and even thicker posterior band (figs 1(*a*)–(*c*)). These characteristics allow the disc to flex as it normalises changes in the interarticular space during chewing. The disc has also been considered to promote lubrication (spreading action), energy absorbtion and joint range of motion.

Synovial cavity and synovium

The synovial cavity is a space of variable extent among individuals. It can be elusive to the inexperienced clinician seeking to inject or aspirate it during treatment. The upper and lower joint cavities are bathed in a viscous synovial fluid secreted by the synovium. This fluid is an ultrafiltrate of blood plasma plus a mucin. It is composed chiefly of highly polymerised hyaluronic acid, which is responsible for the slippery viscous quality.[8] The synovial membrane is the innermost layer of the fibrous capsule and occupies virtually all non-stress-bearing areas within the joint. Unlike the avascular articular tissue, the regenerative capacity of the synovium is excellent. Because the synovial membrane is loose connnective tissue and the synovial cavity arises as a space in connective tissue, it is reasonable to consider this fluid as essentially intercellular material of connective tissue.[8] There is a tendency to consider the function of the synovium one of providing lubrication, but this thin, delicate structure has other functions: nutrition, phagocytosis, and immunological capacity.[9] Material with synovium-like quality also accumulates in tendon sheaths, such as the temporalis tendon sheath. Tendonitis in these sites can be treated in a manner analogous to the treatment of synovitis in the TMJ.

Proliferation of the synovial cells occurs during synovitis, with the concomitant release of prostaglandins and large quantities of collagenase, an enzyme of sparse presence in the normal state.[9] The synovium is normally not very sensitive to pain, so it is reasonable in the clinical setting to attribute pronounced capsular pain and tenderness to the effects of inflammation.

Capsule

The temporomandibular capsule surrounds the joint and unites its parts. Together with the inner synovial layer, its outer, more dense layer is attached to the periphery of the articular disc. The capsule is rather thin, but the lateral surface is strengthened by the lateral ligament which arises from a tubercle on the temporal bone and passes downwards and backwards to the neck of the condyle below the lateral pole.[10] The lateral ligament has two parts, a horizontal band acting to restrict posterior condyle movement, and an oblique band serving to stabilise the joint in translation.[1] Accordingly, these two bands may be put under functional test by retruding the jaw (horizontal band) and by opening widely (oblique band). The sphenomandibular and stylomandibular ligaments are accessory ligaments and have little influence on the movements of the mandible.[1] The compromised joint capsule can be the source of instability or the site of constriction as the condyle attempts to pass over the crest of the articular eminence. The normal joint capsule, however, is well designed to maintain proximity of the joint parts during function. For this reason, attempts to impart involuntary distraction of joint are met with the development of only slight amounts of joint-play in downward or mediolateral planes. Examination of patients and fresh autopsy specimens by this author has dispelled the notion that the normal joint can be grossly distracted in the downward planes. The evaluation and manipulation of joint-play are useful in clinical applications, and will be discussed in Chapters 4 and 7.

Articular disc

Rees's classic article[10] on the mandibular joint called attention to the intricacies of disc structure and function. The disc proper and its attachment tissues are shown in figures 3 and 4. These may be compared with figures 1(a)–(c). The posterior attachment (bilaminar zone) is composed of soft, open-textured tissue containing various amounts of elastin.[11] The increased presence of elastin in the superior lamina is an indication that these tissues are under stretch. The joint is innervated chiefly by the auriculotemporal nerve (trigeminal nerve, mandibular division) via the dorsal aspect of the capsule. The extent and nature of innervation suggest that nociception from compression of the posterior attachment could give rise to painful joint symptoms. While the bilaminar zone described by Rees[10] can be identified, this distinction is mostly limited to the medial half of the joint (fig. 1(c)).[12] The inferior aspect of the posterior attachment (bilaminar zone) has less elastic tissue; it functions to stabilise the disc at the closed position. The medio-lateral disc attachments freely allow antero-

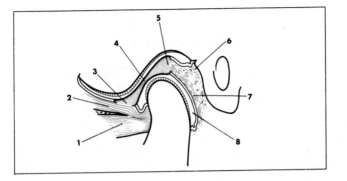

Fig. 3 Sagittal diagram of the medial third of the TMJ depicting the following structures: (1) inferior portion and (2) superior portion of the lateral pterygoid muscle. (3) anterior band; (4) central portion; (5) posterior band of the articular disc; (6) superior lamina of the posterior attachment; (7) inferior lamina of the posterior attachment; (8) lower synovial space. Left side of figure is anterior. Compare with figure 1.

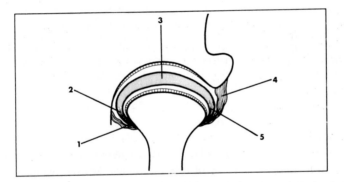

Fig. 4 Frontal diagram of an anteriorly tilted frontal plane through the articular eminence, disc and mandibular condyle, showing the following structures: (1) medial aspect of the capsule; (2) medial discal attachment; (3) central portion of the articular disc; (4) lateral capsule in the area of the lateral ligament; (5) lateral discal attachment, Compare with figure 2.

posterior movement but limit movement in the medio-lateral plane. In the absence of direct trauma, however, displacement of the articular disc is possible only after specific soft tissue changes exist within the joint.

Disc–condyle complex
The articular unit of the lower division of the TMJ is termed the disc–condyle complex.[13] To see why this term is useful, one must consider the nature of the articular interface. Dissimilar convex surfaces of the

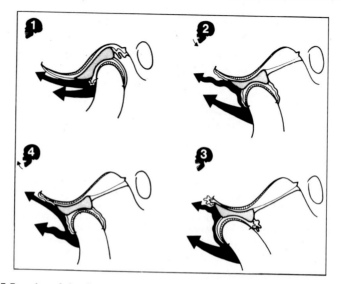

Fig. 5 Function of the disc–condyle complex diagrammed in the sagittal plane. Bold arrows depict the direction and activity in the lateral pterygoid muscle: wavy arrow = less muscular activity; straight arrow = pronounced activity. The functional status of the joint components are shown for different phases of jaw position: (1) closed position; (2) partial opening; (3) full opening; (4) power stroke (partially closed jaw). Note that the activity of the superior portion of the lateral pterygoid muscle is more active on closing than on opening.

temporal and condylar components are stabilised by an articular disc separating the two compartments of the TMJs. It is the intact articular disc that serves as an 'articular surface', with histological structure identical to the fibrous connective tissue of the condyle and articular eminence. The disc has also been stated to be an anatomical prerequisite to this special joint mechanism.[14] It is therefore a misconception to consider the condyle as an element that articulates with the articular eminence.[13]

The disc–condyle complex allows controlled gliding in the upper articular unit, while movement in the lower articular unit is limited largely to hinge movement. The joint is adequately protected to withstand closing movements, but it is subject to injury during sudden transverse force or repetitive lateral thrusts. Under active opening, combined hinge and glide motion are observed, whereas in retrusive jaw manipulation hinge motion is produced.

A recent autopsy study[6] on young adult TMJs was made analogous to that of Rees.[10] The articular surface was seen to be smooth and rounded in TMJs free of articular remodelling. The 'transverse ridge' described by

Rees is undoubtedly a remodelling feature occurring in the changed TMJ. Such formative changes appear to be slightly evident in the condyle in figure 1(*a*). In most cases the superior aspect of the condyle was positioned under the posterior band and central part of the disc, not posterior to it as Rees originally described (see fig. 3). The different findings could be accounted for by differences in age and degree of adaptive changes among the materials of these two studies. Recent arthrographic studies cast doubt on Rees's observation that the 'condylar ridge' slips forward over the disc's anterior band. It is when the joint is unstable that this 'eccentric hinge movement' is seen.

The relationship of the lateral pterygoid muscle to the disc has been somewhat controversial. As can be seen from figures 1(*b*), (*c*) and 3, the superior head of the lateral pterygoid associates with the disc, but mainly inserts in the pterygoid fovea just below the condyle.

Biomechanics of the disc–condyle complex

To appreciate TMJ clicking and restriction fully, it is necessary to understand the basics of disc–condyle function. Hjortsjö's[4,14,15] observations and conclusions of the TMJ mechanism are still valid today. He described the movement of the articular disc as a rotation about a centre passing through the articular eminence, with simultaneous motion of the condyle about its horizontal axis. Hjortsjö likened the TMJ to a biaxial nutcracker. The status of the disc at various phases of jaw movement is shown in figure 5. This figure and the following description are intended to augment and clarify the fundamental contributions of Rees.[10]

Opening phase

During opening, the articular disc rotates posteriorly about the condyle as the disc–condyle complex moves forward and downward about the articular eminence. The build-up of tension in the posterior attachment at mid-opening helps bring backward disc rotation about the condyle. Inactivity in the superior part of the lateral pterygoid muscle during opening[16] facilitates this action. Hence, it is unlikely that the lateral pterygoid plays a strong role in pulling the disc forward during opening, as has been implied.[10] The often described 'recoil' action of the posterior attachment during jaw closing is relatively unimportant compared with its influence on the disc during jaw opening. During the mid-range of opening, the joint remains passive and unstressed.

Full opening

At full opening, gliding of the disc is nullified by the limitations of muscle stretch, resistance in the capsule, and by the lack of available articular surface. Exaggerated jaw opening movement beyond this point causes subluxation, such as uneven, jerky movement of the disc–condyle complex over the non-articular surfaces. When the mouth is fully opened, the soft tissue is sucked in from the postero-lateral aspects of the joint.[10]

Power stroke

In the closing or power stroke, the joint receives maximum stress. At this point sudden distracting forces on the condyle are produced by the resistance of the bolus of food. Activity in the superior part of the lateral pterygoid muscle on closing[14] provides an anterior component of tension on the disc and causes the disc to move forward. In this instance, the disc functions as a 'moving wedge' to insure full contact between the joint components during maximum function. The integrity of the posterior band therefore prevents anterior displacement of the disc during normal function.

Occlusal position

At full closure, the disc is rotated forward with its surfaces in a close-packed* joint relationship. The disc is stabilised at this point by the build-up of tension in the inferior lamina of the posterior attachment, lateral ligament and by the passive effects of disc form. This perspective of disc mechanics should be remembered when the clinical implications of TMJ pathofunction are discussed in a subsequent paper.

Radiological aspects of clinical interest

Radiography of the TMJ has always been technically difficult. This obstacle has been exacerbated by the lack of agreement as to the usefulness of the findings, which until recently have been limited to observation of the osseous parts. The lack of agreement between TMJ radiographic changes and TM pain and dysfunction is the centre of the controversy. Both under-diagnosis and over-diagnosis are everyday risks. It is not so much due to a lack of technical knowledge and diagnostic understanding as it is the lack of application of this knowledge which has been developed over the last thirty years.

In a relatively short time, many advances have been forthcoming. Since

---

*The joint surface becomes fully congruent.

1980 arthrography of the TMJ has become common, and newer imaging systems such as computer-aided tomography (CAT) and nuclear magnetic resonance (NMR) offer promises of readily exposing the soft tissues of the TMJ for diagnostic evaluation. Arthroscopic procedures, particularly those employed therapeutically, are already being investigated world wide.

Technical considerations

Radiography of the TMJ is frustrating because of the joint's position relative to bony masses in the skull, notably the petrous ridge. To deal with this, plain radiography techniques such as the transcranial lateral oblique projection were developed, despite the fact that this projection yielded a distorted image. Moreover, the resultant image was limited to an appreciation of the lateral aspect of the condyle with lesser information as to condyle position and articular eminence morphology. Palla[17] has reviewed the salient technical and diagnostic standards for this projection, which still deserve a place in TMJ radiography.

Tomography is body section radiography. Tomography has become the standard for comprehensive evaluation of the bony components of the TMJ, mostly because it allows visualisation of the temporal and condylar component. In addition, it allows the best evaluation of condyle position.[18] Interpretation of a technically correct tomogram is straightforward because its projection can be viewed in standard anatomical planes. Despite its many advantages, full capability tomographic equipment is expensive to use, although moderately expensive linear tomographic systems have been employed extensively within the past few years.

Both tomographic and plain projections have distortion effects if the angles of the x-ray beam are not related to the horizontal axis of the condyle and mandibular fossa. Hence a cephalostat or fluoroscopic orientation of the x-ray beam is required. Unfortunately, many radiologists in hospitals have not had sufficient clinical motivation to raise their standards to this level of sophistication.

The following radiological principles should be kept in mind. Projections should be taken in two or more planes. Axial correction should be made of the condylar axis by the use of preliminary basilar projections followed by orientation with a cephalostat. Cephalostats are particularly useful because they permit reproducible views over time. With tomography, sagittal closed views should be taken in the medial, central and lateral parts of the joint. Most importantly, the views taken should represent maxillomandibular positions of clinical relevance. Lastly, all radiographic examinations should have the benefit of a written interpretation.

Representative sagittal tomograms are shown in figure 6(a)–(c). These projections in the central plane represent a focal thickness of tissue of from 4 to 8 mm, which explain the double images seen in some views. The frontal view (fig. 6(d)) is most valuable in demonstrating condylar remodelling and other changes. It is taken by tilting the head backward 10°, whilst the jaw is protruded; frontal plane projections are then made and the best obtainable cut is accepted for interpretation.[16]

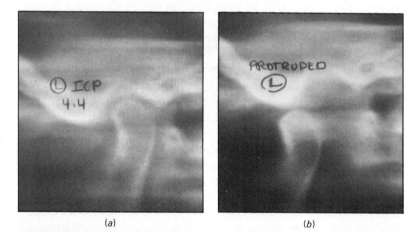

(a)   (b)

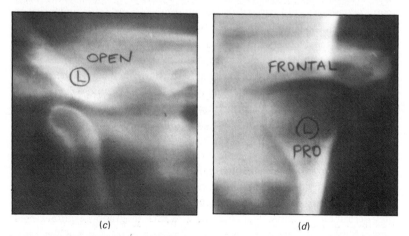

(c)   (d)

Fig. 6 (a,b,c) Linear tomograms taken in the lateral plane and (d) frontal plane in the following maxillomandibular positions: (a) intercuspal position. (b) protruded position. (c) full open position. (d) protruded position. All views show the middle portion of the joint. L: Left joint, from the side (a-c) and front (d).

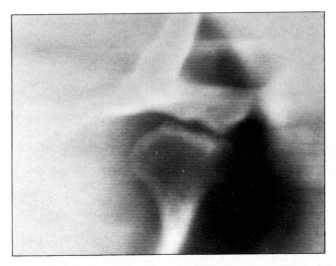

Fig. 7 Linear tomogram of a patient with troublesome joint noise and discomfort taken in the frontal plane with the jaw in a protruded position. Note gross arthrotic changes in the lateral half of the articular eminence and condyle revealed by this projection.

Figure 7 demonstrates an example of a frontal projection showing marked remodelling of the condyle in a patient complaining of troublesome joint noise and discomfort. Often these changes are not well identified in sagittal projections.

The following tomographic views are recommended: closed sagittal views (medial, central, lateral cut), protruded and maximally open sagittal view (central cut only), frontal plane view with the jaw in protrusion (central cut only), and panoramic survey of the jaw region. Modern high quality x-ray equipment combined with the use of rare earth intensifying screens has rendered the delivered radiation dose to approximately that of a full mouth dental radiographic series.

Indications

It has always been a rule that the decision to order radiographs should be made in anticipation that they could very likely influence the proposed treatment and prognosis. Having this in mind, radiographs of the TMJ should be considered mostly for cases where the cause of pain and dysfunction cannot be understood or where conservative short-term care does not alleviate the symptoms.

In a sense, the decision to do TMJ radiographs will vary depending upon the highest degree of understanding of the clinician. The more definitive the examination, history and clinical diagnosis, the fewer surprises there will be from the radiographic survey. Other screening projections such as panoramic view may suffice to rule out observable causes of TMJ pain and dysfunction.

This author has progressively ordered fewer radiographs as his experience in diagnosing TMJ pathology has given increasing competence. It is not consistent with good patient management to subject all patients complaining of various signs and symptoms of TM disorders to radiographic procedures. However, to ignore the diagnostic indications for TMJ radiograms on selected patients is equally untenable.

Acknowledgements

Research reported by the author was supported by a National Institute of Dental Research Grant, Number ROIDE-05381-3. Irene Petrovicius of UCLA Dental Illustration and Rhoda Freeman of the Word Processing Center at UCLA School of Dentistry are thanked for their services.

References

1 Sicher H and DuBrul E L. *Oral anatomy,* 6th ed, pp 160–191. St Louis: C V Mosby, 1975.
2 Williams P L, Warwick R. *Gray's anatomy,* 36th ed, p 429. Edinburgh: Churchill Livingstone, 1980.
3 Wright D M, Moffett B C Jr. The postnatal development of the human temporomandibular joint. *Am J Anat* 1974; **141:** 235–249.
4 Hjortsjö C-H, Persson P-I, Sonesson B. Studies on the shape of the articular eminence with its relation to the mechanism in the temporomandibular joint. *Odontologisk Revy* 1953; **4:** 187–202.
5 Yoon C, Nordström B, Hansson T L, Solberg W K, Forsythe A. A quantitative method for condylar form analysis. *J Dent Res* 1984; **63:** Abstr No. 520, p 228.
6 Solberg W K, Hansson T L, Nordström B N. The temporomandibular joint in young adults at autopsy: a morphologic classification and evaluation. *J Oral Rehab* 1985; **12:** 303–321.
7 Hansson T, Öberg T, Carlsson G E, Kopp S. Thickness of the soft tissue layers and the articular disc in the temporomandibular joint. *Acta Odontol Scand* 1977; **35:** 77–83.
8 Wilson F C. *The musculoskeletal system: basic processes and disorders,* 2nd ed, pp 210. Philadelphia: Lippincott, 1983.
9 Angus B. Joints in general. *In* Friedman M H, Weisberg J (eds). *Temporomandibular joint disorders, diagnosis and treatment,* p 12. Chicago: Quintessence, 1985.
10 Rees L A. The structure and function of the mandibular joint. *Br Dent J* 1954; **96:** 125–133.
11 Dixon A D. Structure and functional significance of the intra-articular disc of the human temporomandibular joint. *Oral Surg* 1962; **15:** 48–61.
12 Ridall E R, Hayes E R, Tamburlin J H, Tabak L A, Mohl N D. Description of elastic fibers in the bilaminar zone. *J Dent Res* 1982; **61:** Abstr No. 1554, p 1551.
13 Bell W E. Understanding temporomandibular biomechanics. *J Craniomandibular Practice* 1983; **1:** 27–33.

14 Hjortsjö C-H. The significance of the articular disc and the 'accentuated grinding joint'. *Odont Revy* 1953; **4:** 203–209.

15 Hjortsjö C-H. An apparatus illustrating the mechanism in the temporomandibular joint. *Odontologisk Revy* 1953; **4:** 93–106.

16 Mahan P A, Gibbs C J and Mauderli A. Superior and inferior lateral pterygoid activity (abstract). *J Dent Res* 1982; **61:** 272.

17 Palla S. Condyle position: Determinants and radiological analysis. *In* Solberg W K, Clark G T (eds). *Abnormal jaw mechanics: diagnosis and treatment*, pp 51–76. Chicago: Quintessence, 1984.

18 Blaschke D D. Temporomandibular joint. *In* Goaz P, White S (eds). *Oral radiology: principles and interpretation*, pp 508–601. St Louis: C V Mosby, 1982.

3 Clinical significance of TMJ changes

Adaptive processes associated with temporomandibular (TM) disorders are brought about by the shifting equilibrium between form and function. When functional demands on the temporomandibular joint (TMJ) increase, there is a compensatory shift in order to cope with the details of articular fit and function.[1] Structural and functional alterations of the articular tissues, such as articular remodelling, are apparent before symptoms are evident, continue during the clinical phases of TM disorders, and persist in the degenerative phase of osteoarthrosis.

In light of this, the clinician should not consider TM disorders as 'all or none' conditions but should consider the natural changes involved in their progression and regression. The TM disorder occurs when normal protective processes become decompensated, or when they are abruptly altered, as in the case of macrotrauma. Articular remodelling, disc displacement, deformation of the disc, loosening or tightening of the capsule, alteration of condyle position, and degenerative changes are among the potential findings which may be evaluated. The most effective treatments are those that increase the capacity for recuperative processes to achieve a natural equilibrium.[1]

The purpose of this paper is to review articular changes associated with TM disorders and to discuss the implications of these changes for patient management.

Articular remodelling
Articular remodelling is accomplished through a cellular response to

biomechanical stress. It serves to maintain the equilibrium between joint form and function; as such it is physiological, not pathological.[2] These changes are first characterised by a thickening of the cartilage zone (fig. 1) of the articular tissue. This thickening correlates with a significant depletion of the mesenchymal cells of the proliferation zone (fig. 1).[3] These histological changes in the soft tissues are later accompanied by radiographically visible changes in the bony contours. The disc, having no undifferentiated mesenchyme, does not appear to undergo active remodelling: it passively deforms by physical compression to accommodate changes in the temporal and condylar components.[1] If functional demands exceed the capacity of this protective mechanism, the balance between form and function shifts over to a pathological state and the cellular responses taken on a destructive character referred to as osteoarthrosis (OA).[1] Osteoarthrosis is therefore a breakdown or loss of articular tissue, resulting in friction and disc perforation. It should be noted that the articular zone of tissue (most superficial) (fig. 1) and the disc do not appear to participate in the remodelling process except by passive accommodation to changes elsewhere in the temporal and condylar components.

The contours of the joint continue to change throughout life as a result of articular remodelling. The grossly visible evidence of remodelling is termed deviation in form (DIF).[3] These surface irregularities appear as

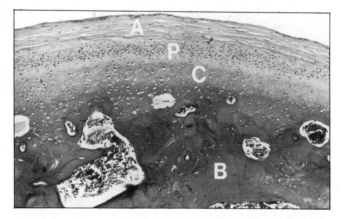

Fig. 1 Light-microscopy sagittal section through the lateral aspect of the human mandibular condyle from a 20-year-old female. The following layers of articular tissue may be identified: A, articular zone; P, proliferative zone; C, cartilagenous zone; B, bone. This specimen is free of remodelling changes. (From Solberg W K and Hansson T L, unpublished material, Temporomandibular Joint Laboratory, UCLA Dental Research Institute, Los Angeles, Ca.)

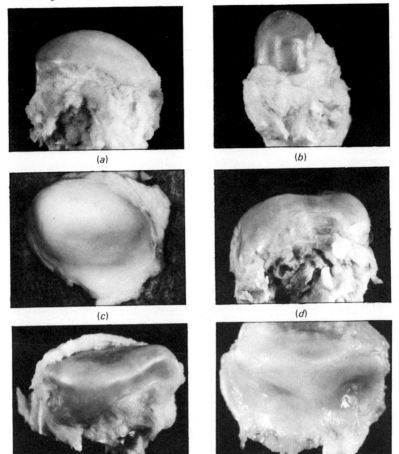

Fig. 2 Freely dissected human mandibular condyles and articular discs from young adults. (a)-(c) Unchanged left mandibular condyle and articular disc from a 27-year-old female.

(a) Anterior aspect of condyle;

(b) Medial aspect of condyle;

(c) Articular disc from above, anterior band at bottom;

(d-e) Left mandibular condyle and articular disc from a 23-year-old male displaying extensive deviation in form (DIF);

(d) Anterior aspect of condyle;

(e) Condyle from above, lateral pole to the right;

(f) Articular disc from above revealing localised DIF, anterior band at the bottom.

(From Solberg W K, Hansson T L, Norstrom B. The temporomandibular joint in young adults at autopsy: a morphologic classification and evaluation. *J Oral Rehab* 1985; **12**: 303-321.)

flattened, elevations on the temporal and condylar components and by the passive thinning of the articular disc. Examples of DIF on the mandibular condyle and articular disc are shown in figure 2(d)-(f) in comparison with examples free of these changes (fig. 2(a)-(c). The distribution of these changes in autopsy material[4] derived from 51 young adults is shown in figure 3. The location of these juxtaposed changes in functional areas of the articular surface suggests that they are responses to functional stimuli. DIF was common in the majority of joints, and in one-third of these cases all joint components were affected at least to some degree. The component most often found to have extensive DIF was the condyle. Arthrosis, on the other hand, was observed only on the articular eminence and articular disc.[4]

Clinical significance

A feature of the TMJ with advanced changes is the finding of exuberant remodelling of the condyle in combination with degenerative changes in the temporal bone and disc.[5] Radiographic overinterpretation frequently occurs when condylar changes are considered to be evidence of arthrosis when in fact they are most likely to represent pre-arthrotic bony remodelling. This is particularly common when the transcranial radiograph is used because it fails to reveal early changes in the temporal bone. Therefore differentiation between remodelling and osteoarthrosis is tenuous when using radiographic results alone.

Clicking and incoordination in the TMJ can be explained in part by functional interference created when remodelling achieves sufficient extent and bulk. The radiographic diagnosis should therefore include an account of these changes, particularly in the light of progressive clinical symptoms. For example, the clicking joint with extensive DIF is probably not going to respond to therapy in the same manner as those joints free of radiographic changes.

Condyle shape

Condyle shape continues to be an important factor in radiographic interpretation, but the implications of individual shape characteristics are largely unknown. A classification of condyle shapes in young adults is shown in figure 4. Younger joints had a more even curvature of their silhouettes than has been previously suggested.[4] Condyles with few or no DIFs were more often slightly rounded, convex, or elliptical in their respective planes, whereas condyles with DIF were relatively more gable shaped, or cylindrical and irregular in appearance (fig. 4).

The condyle and temporal component showed inter-relationships of

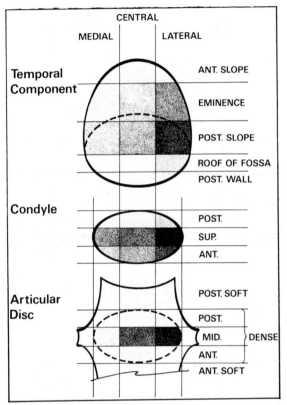

Fig. 3 Distribution of DIF among the TMJ components. The intensity of stippling is proportional to the frequency of DIF occurring in each sector. The most common sites for DIF are on functionally related areas. (Same credits as in figure 2.)

shapes, particularly for those features that might be considered most optimal because of their negative association with DIF (fig. 5).[4] Applied in diagnosis, the above insights are useful in judging radiographic shapes among individuals of varying age and oral function. In broad terms, condylar shape is functionally linked with geometric alterations of the whole ramus during growth and maintenance.[6]

Displacement of the articular disc

The position of the articular disc has received a great deal of attention in connection with internal derangement of the TMJ. Although displacement of the articular disc in young individuals with internal derangement of the TMJ has been established by arthrography, the clinical context of these findings failed to clarify whether these changes might also occur as

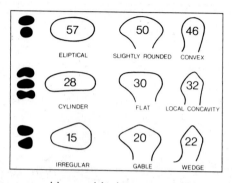

Fig. 4 Classification summarising condyle shapes among 95 young adults, mean age 26·4 ± 6·8 years. Percentages are given for each category. The ellipsoid shape is characteristic of the growing condyle which may undergo alterations in shape during late growth and maturity. Departure from ellipsoid shape was associated with those condyles displaying extensive DIF. (Same credits as in figure 1.)

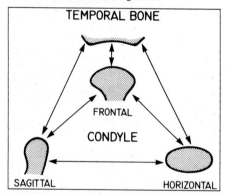

Fig. 5 The most significant interrelationships of condylar and temporal component shapes with respect to plane of reference. *Arrows* indicate that positive relationships exist among all classified shapes shown above. (Same credits as in figure 2.)

incidental findings.

In a recent study[4] of 95 unselected young adult TMJs, the position of the articular disc was classified according to the relationship of the superior crest of the condyle to the posterior band of the disc (fig. 6). Partial or total displacement of the articular disc were identified in 12% of the joints, 7% partial and 4% total. Most of the displacements were in the anteriomedial direction. A striking finding was the greater frequency and severity of disc displacement among female specimens.[4] Unfortunately, no data were available to judge the extent to which these displacements might have caused clinical problems. These findings may explain, at least in part, why

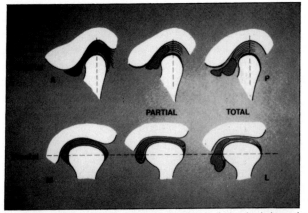

Fig. 6 Classification of the position of the articular disc. In the sagittal plane, the posterior band of the disc is usually centred over the superior crest of the condyle, upper left view. In the frontal plane, the lateral dense part of the disc is usually located at the lateral pole, lower left view. Partial displacement, middle views. Total displacement, right views.

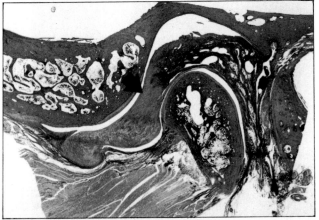

Fig. 7 Sagittal section through the medial aspect of a human temporomandibular joint from a 33-year-old female with an excellent Angle Class I dentition. The articular disc was totally displaced. *Arrow* indicates metaplastic changes in the area of the posterior attachment; this tissue appears to have been converted into a dense pad resembling the disc proper. (Same credits as in figure 1.)

more women in the USA and Scandinavia have TMJ surgery with the aim of ameliorating clinical TMJ derangement.

What is the destiny of the disc once it is displaced? The findings from anatomical studies shed some light on this question. Figure 7 shows a specimen where the disc is totally displaced. Close examination reveals that the posterior attachment (arrow) has been in a zone of repetitive loading.

The expected open-textured architecture of the posterior attachment of the disc now appears to be a dense pad resembling the disc proper. The posterior attachment has evidently undergone metaplasia, a process whereby the conversion of one form of connective tissue into another occurs in response to a changing stimulus. In short, the joint in figure 7 is

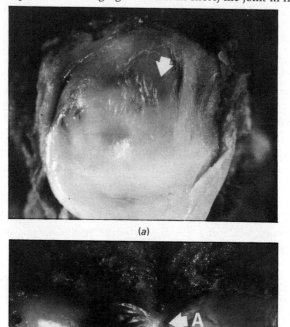

(a)

(b)

Fig. 8 Partially displaced articular disc from the right temporomandibular joint of a 30-year-old male with bilateral loss of posterior tooth support, superior view. (a) Ruggedness (*arrow*) can be seen in the posterior band of the articular disc. Lateral towards the left, posterior towards the top. (b) Same joint as in (a), showing superior aspect of the condyle and the inferior surface of the disc still joined to the condyle by the medial disc attachment (letter A). Note mediolateral ridge (R) traversing the usually smooth middle part of the disc. (Same credits as figure 2.)

an example of the compromises that nature arranges to cope with abrupt morphological alterations.

The disc shown in figure 8(a)–(b) was found to be partially displaced, a finding not uncommon to surgeons who open the TMJs. In this specimen, the posterior band of the articular disc has apparently undergone deformation due to functional stresses (fig. 8(a)). It is rugged and thinned (arrow), and it has lost its ability to serve as a functional wedge. The underside of the disc is ridged in a medio-lateral direction, and this thickness is now observed where the thin central part of the disc would normally be found (fig. 8(b)). This ridge would seem to limit the mobility of the disc-condyle complex.

Clinical implications

Changes in disc position and shape occur through the mechanism of accommodative displacement, as compared with the resistive toughening and thickening characteristic of articular remodelling. The system accommodates to this change by conversion of once vascularised non-articular tissue into more dense articular tissue. The message here is clear. While the phenomenon of disc displacement is not normal, it is neither wholly pathological. Clinically, many people survive displacements of discs without long term problems,[7] provided the forces directed to non-articular tissues do not exceed the joint's ability to undergo metaplasia without inflammation. If the clicking or locking TMJ cannot be completely normalised, clinical efforts should be directed toward decreasing loading to the joints during the most troublesome episodes.

Condyle position

Radiographic condyle position and its role in TMJ pathology have been discussed for over the last thirty years. Abnormal forward position of one or both condyles has been associated with Angle Class II malocclusions and dual bite.

True condylar distractions and fulcruming of the mandibular condyles have been associated with open bites. Superior condyle positioning with decreased joint space is a classic radiographic sign associated with TMJ osteoarthrosis or acute trauma to the articular disc.

Although atypical condyle positions and their relationship to skeletal and dento-alveolar abnormalities have been acknowledged, abnormal retropositioning of the condyle and its relationship to oral rehabilitation have continued to be controversial (fig. 9). The controversy is now beginning to be addressed with the introduction of better radiographic

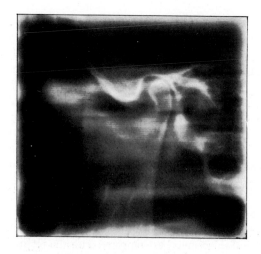

Fig. 9 Linear tomogram showing marked retropositioning of the mandibular condyle.

techniques and interpretation. Unfortunately, radiology of the TMJ is a complex procedure for which many clinicians are ill equipped. Under optimal conditions, both tomographic[8] and plain transcranial techniques[9] are useful in the interpretation of condyle position.

Abnormal condyle retroposition has been associated with TM disorders,[8-10] but different methods and instrumentation made the results difficult to compare. Recent tomographic studies by Pullinger *et al.*[10] have confirmed that patients with TMJ derangement (clicking and locking joint) have significantly more condylar retropositioning than a asymptomatic comparison group. Women controls had more condylar retropositioning than men, possibly due to a recognised predisposition of women toward hypermobility and joint instability.[11] In summary, mild retrocondylar positioning is a passive factor in women controls and a factor common to both men and women suffering from TMJ derangement. However, in view of the substantial range of variability observed in condyle position, the diagnosis of TMJ dysfunction cannot be based solely upon radiographic observation of non-concentricity.[8]

Joint laxity

The term joint laxity indicates a tendency toward hypermobility. Increased laxity in the TMJ may lead to functional instability and soreness.[11] An important manifestation of TMJ laxity is open dislocation (luxation). There is controversy over why this occurs, but there is general agreement that

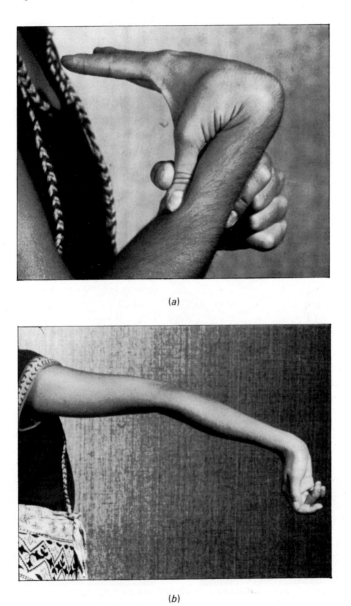

(a)

(b)

Fig. 10 Examination of a young woman with hypermobility of wrists, fingers (a) and elbow (b) in association with internal derangement of the right temporomandibular joint. Joint laxity is common in young women.[1]

laxity of capsular structures are involved. Examination of the wrists, fingers and elbows (fig. 10(a)-(b)) for hyperextension, particularly in tall young girls, may reveal that benign hyperlaxity is a generalised joint problem. This worsens the prognosis for therapy directed exclusively to the TMJ. Laxity is more common in women and may predispose them to more symptoms. Joint laxity may be a cause for joint clicking. Therefore, open stretch therapy is not recommended for persons with joint clicking. A fundamental goal in treatment of laxity is to control forces which put the joints on excessive tension or shear. Limitation of functional demands, neuromuscular training and functional alignment of the occlusion are means to this end.

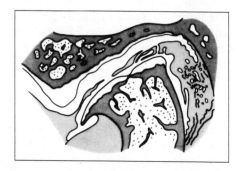

Fig. 11 Drawing of a temporomandibular joint with osteoarthrosis. Marked degenerative changes are portrayed including an eroded articular eminence, remnants of the articular disc, degenerated articular surface of the condyle with osteophyte. (From Mahan P E, The temporomandibular joint in function and pathofunction. *In* Solberg W K and Clark G T (eds) *Temporomandibular joint problems, biologic diagnosis and treatment.* pp 33-49. Chicago: Quintessence, 1980.)

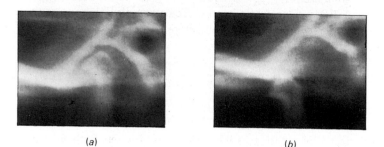

(a)   (b)

Fig. 12 Linear tomograms, lateral view of patient with osteoarthritis, displaying the radiographic equivalent of the changes shown in figure 11. (a) Closed mouth view; (b) open mouth view.

Osteoarthrosis

Articular remodelling is a biological mechanism that serves to maintain an equilibrium between joint form and function.[2] When this defence mechanism is overwhelmed, the non-vascularised articular tissue becomes injured without pain and inflammation.[1] Remodelling continues, but within the larger context of pathological tissue destruction. This process is termed osteoarthrosis (OA). To understand the process of tissue degeneration, we should regard it conceptually as the destruction of articular tissue that begins whenever the contours of a joint have not adapted successfully to the functional or other forces imposed upon it.[1]

Osteoarthrosis is most often asymptomatic, but when symptoms develop, they are usually mechanical, involving interference, friction, or restriction. Synovitis is often seen as a clinical complication and will be covered in a subsequent paper in this series. It has been suggested that the definition of OA be broadened to include the degenerative changes of the deeper zones of the articular cartilage and the subchondral bone occurring simultaneously with a microscopically intact articular surface.[12] In OA, deterioration occurs by disruption of the collagen fibre network and fatty degeneration.[13] Generally, the term OA is meant to imply the destruction of articular tissue and bone (figs 11 and 12(*a*)-(*b*)). Not all parts of the joint are affected equally. Osteoarthrosis commences first on the temporal eminence and in the lateral part of the disc and is seen in the condyle and in the medial parts of the joint under more extensive involvement.[5] Once the degenerative process is under way, healing may occur in early and moderate stages only when the capacity for cellular remodelling is increased by therapy or as the demands on the joint are decreased.[1]

It is assumed that the cause of this wear and tear is mechanical, resulting either from excessive repetitive loading or from the functional capacity of the joint being reduced by other host factors. Displacement of the articular disc is a common finding (64%) at autopsies on randomly selected elderly individuals[12] and more common than in young adults.[4] In the majority of cases, OA and disc displacement were observed in the same individuals.[12] This association suggests that disc displacement, like progressive and regressive remodelling, is one of the accompanying signs of OA. In this connection, Moffett[1] has aptly stated that OA (degenerative joint disease) is the final common pathway for all diseases, injuries and derangements that affect a joint during its life cycle. This view sets forth an important clinical perspective. The onset of OA is a result of an inadequate articular remodelling response and not the result of spontaneous events. Awareness that the threshold between remodelling and tissue degeneration is reversible in early stages of the disease directs the clinician to focus his efforts toward reversing this progressive process.

Conclusion

Too often, TMJ disorders have been identified as disturbances of function without due consideration to the structural alterations that, according to biological laws, normally occur in association with dysfunction. In the past, emphasis on 'neuromuscular TMJ problems' implied that functional factors, including functional pain, were the only mechanisms involved in TM disorders. To claim that organic features of TM disorders have been excluded simply after routine radiographic examination is simplistic.[5] Awareness of TMJ changes discussed in this paper provides a more realistic perspective than the commonly stated belief that TMJ problems are merely states of dysfunction and do not involve organic changes.

References

1 Moffett B C. Definitions of temporomandibular joint derangements. *In* Moffett B C (ed). *Diagnosis of internal derangements of the temporomandibular joint Vol. 1: Double-contrast arthrography and clinical correlation.* pp 6–7. Seattle: University of Washington Continuing Dental Education, 1984.

2 Moffett B C, Johnson L C, McCabe J B, Askew H C. Articular remodeling in the adult human temporomandibular joint. *Am J Anat* 1964; **115:** 119–130.

3 Hansson T L, Öberg T. Arthrosis and deviation in form in the temporomandibular joint. A macroscopic study on a human autopsy material. *Acta Odont Scand* 1977; **35:** 167–174.

4 Solberg W K, Hansson T L, Nordström B. The temporomandibular joint in young adults at autopsy: a morphologic classification and evaluation. *J Oral Rehab* 1985; **12:** 303–321.

5 Carlsson G E, Kopp S, Öberg T. Arthritis and allied diseases of the temporomandibular joint. *In* Zarb G A, Carlsson G E (eds) *Temporomandibular joint function and dysfunction.* pp 269–320. Copenhagen: Munksgaard, 1979.

6 Mack P J. A functional explanation for the morphology of the temporomandibular joint of man. *J Dent* 1984; **12:** 225–230.

7 Mejersjö C, Carlsson G E. Long term results of treatment for temporomandibular pain and dysfunction. *J Prosthet Dent* 1983; **49:** 809–815.

8 Pullinger A G, Hollender L, Solberg W K, Petersson A. A tomographic study of mandibular condyle position in an asymptomatic population. *J Prosthet Dent* 1985; **53:** 706–713.

9 Palla S. Condyle position: Determinants and radiological analysis. *In* Solberg W K, Clark G T (eds). *Abnormal jaw mechanics: diagnosis and treatment.* pp 51–76. Chicago: Quintessence, 1984.

10 Pullinger A G, Solberg W K, Hollender L, Guichet D. Tomographic analysis of mandibular condyle position of diagnostic subgroups in temporomandibular disorders. *J Prosthet Dent* 1986; **55:** 723–729.

11 Beighton P, Grahame R, Bird Q. *Hypermobility of joints,* pp 39. New York: Springer-Verlag, 1983.

12 De Bont L G M, Boering G, Liem R S B, Eulderink F, Westersson P L. Osteoarthrosis and internal derangement of the temporomandibular joint. A light microscopic study. Unpublished data.

13 De Bont L G M, Boering G, Liem R S B, Havinga P. Osteoarthritis of the temporomandibular joint: A light microscopic and scanning electron microscopic study of the articular cartilage of the mandibular condyle. *J Oral Maxillofac Surg* 1985; **43:** 481–488.

4 Physical tests in diagnosis

Temporomandibular (TM) disorders represent a curious combination of psychological and somatic manifestations, yet the inclusion criteria[1] for the 'case definition' are dependent upon physical findings. The signature of the TM disorder is pain provoked by function. Moreover, pain and dysfunction go hand in hand. Proper diagnosis is therefore dependent upon a thorough examination in accordance with standards developed for other acquired soft tissue injuries or disorders that result in musculoskeletal or neuromuscular pain and dysfunction. As stated by Cailliet,[2] 'the examination must specifically test the motion of the joint and musculature and expectantly reproduce the specific symptoms'.

The goals of functional testing for soft tissue disorders are twofold: (1) to test the adequacy of the moving part; and (2) to provoke the symptoms and thereby gain awareness of the mechanism of the pain or dysfunction.[2] The physical tests and measures consist of active range of motion (AROM), passive range of motion (PROM), TMJ manipulation, loading tests on the muscles and the joints, and palpation for muscle and joint tenderness. Diagnostic analgesic injections are occasionally employed to identify the source of pain. It should be noted that psychometric tests, radiographs, and the identification of occlusal interferences play a lesser role in the differential diagnosis of TM disorders.

Far too often, diverse chronic sensory disorders of the head and neck have been included under the diagnosis of 'TMJ' with consequent problems in management. The purpose of this article is to suggest how the clinician may absolutely identify TM disorders by objective means, or alternatively, to rule out masticatory disorders as the cause of head and jaw pain or dysfunction. The premise underlying this approach is that TM pain usually relates reasonably well with the demands of function and therefore functional testing will yield diagnostic rewards.

Range of motion

The magnitude and quality of mandibular movements in all planes are usually the best objective indicators of temporo-mandibular joint (TMJ) and masticatory muscle status. Since ROM can be accurately reproduced, an improvement in this finding is a bona fide signal that the pain and dysfunction are moving towards normalisation. Despite the attention usually given to the magnitude and path of mouth opening, the patient's self-report as to the presence and exact location of pain, stiffness or restriction during movement, is equally informative.

Active range of motion

Active range of motion (AROM) denotes that the patient is opening under voluntary effort (fig. 1). There can be restriction (hypomobility) or excessive movement (hypermobility). Limitation of AROM is associated with pain, TMJ internal derangement or neuromuscular disorders. Hypermobility is caused by joint laxity and instability in the disc–condyle complex and capsule. Alterations in AROM are not specific for joint or muscle restriction; this distinction can be achieved by evaluating PROM.[3]

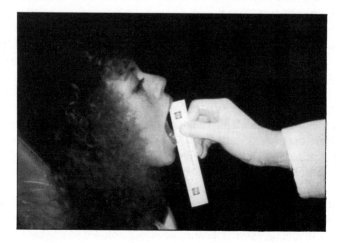

Fig. 1 Active range of motion (AROM).

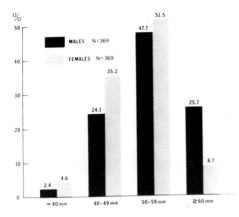

Fig. 2 Active range of motion summarised for 739 otherwise normal young adults. The mean interincisal opening for women (50·9 mm, SD = 6·74) was different from that for men (54·4 mm, SD = 7·14 mm, $P<0·05$).

Men open more widely than women[4] (fig. 2) but the distribution of AROM is relatively consistent from the early teens to old age.[4-5] A 40 mm interincisal opening is a realistic lower limit for persons from 10 to 70 years of age. Agerberg[6] has shown that the chance of observing an interincisal opening of 40 mm or less in healthy young adults is approximately 2%. Therefore, variation from normal AROM (fig. 2), even without pain, may imply possible dysfunction and disease. Conversely, as pointed out by Hansson and Nilner,[7] many patients with dysfunction have mouth openings greater than 40 mm.

In the context of screening, abnormal AROM is rather infrequent.[4] Nevertheless, the association of restricted opening with other frequently observed signs and symptoms indicates that it is an extremely useful contribution to clinical diagnosis (fig. 3).

Passive range of motion

Passive range of motion (PROM) indicates that the examiner moves the part while the patient's musculature is relaxed (fig. 4). The attempt is made to eliminate muscle action; the muscles are 'passive' and are not being evaluated. If AROM is painful while PROM is not, suspect the source of the pain to be in the muscle.[3]

Limited PROM suggests joint dysfunction or mechanical muscle conditions such as TMJ adhesions or muscular contracture. Passive range of motion will be characterised by a 'hard' end feel suggestive of adhesion, arthrosis, or contracture. Increased opening or a 'springy' end feel under

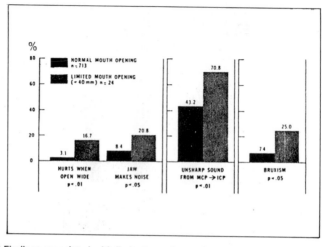

Fig. 3 Findings associated with limited mouth opening. Unsharp sounds from MCP to ICP refer to the quality of occlusal sounds during slow, deliberate tapping of the teeth.

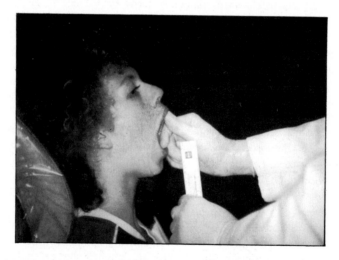

Fig. 4 Passive range of motion (PROM) performed by the examiner

passive stretch suggests neuromuscular restriction. This finding is due to muscular splinting (reflex muscle hyperactivity). If the end feel is abrupt at approximately 26 mm with a history of the jaw 'going out', consider manipulative reduction (see below). Increased ROM from reductive manipulation suggests locking due to displacement of the articular disc.

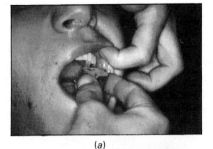

(a)

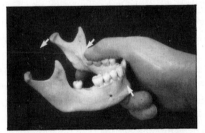

(b)

(c)

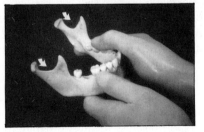

(d)

Fig. 5 Manipulative reduction of the articular disc in the locking patient: (a) preliminary distraction by biting on cork; (b) manual distraction of the joint under active thrusting by the patient; (c) downward and backward pressure on the molars with upward pressure in the chin region; (d) forward and contralateral guided movement.

TMJ manipulation

Sudden onset of jaw restriction, known as locking, can be experienced by the individual with a chronically clicking TMJ. Locking can also be the first sign of joint instability that is later followed by chronic clicking. Locking is characterised by an irreducible anteromedially displaced articular disc. Usually it is evident on one side at a time. Generally this takes place without undue pain. Typically the patient will complain that 'my joint used to click but now it won't open all the way and it doesn't click anymore'.

Reductive manipulation is a technique whereby the examiner causes involuntary condylar distraction followed by protrusive and contralateral guided thrusts (figs 5 (a)-(d)). This is a diagnostic technique that will serve as treatment.[8] If the restriction is due to acute disc displacement, this manoeuvre will be rewarded by an immediate increase in AROM, usually up to or beyond normal limits. The diagnostic value of this procedure is obvious. It is far better to explain these events using orthopaedic explanations rather than to send the patient away with the usual counselling about the need for stress relaxation and muscle relaxant remedies.

Diagnostic advantages aside, the value of this technique is that it is often urgently needed as a therapeutic measure. This is evident by the findings that chronic inflammatory processes often accompany the displaced disc that remains unreduced.[8] The procedure is as follows: (1) place a prop on the affected side and have the patient bite firmly for five minutes (fig. 5 (a)); (2) remove the prop and manually exert downward pressure on the second molar with simultaneous upward pressure in the region of the mentum (fig. 5 (b)); (3) instruct the patient to move forward and then to the opposite side in deliberate sequence whilst the examiner maintains distracting pressure on the moving joint (figs 5 (c) and (d)). There is the impression that great force is necessary to accomplish disc reduction, but this is not so. When successful, this procedure should be followed by the immediate placement of a temporary bite appliance which positions the mandible anteriorly. The attempt is to 'splint' the injured joint orthopaedically in a stable disc–condyle relationship.

Resistance tests

If a masticatory muscle disorder involves a significant amount of muscle mass, application of maximal resistance directed to that muscle will provoke a feeling of pain or an ache. In the correct procedure, muscle function is initiated by passive resistance of the examiner while the joint is maintained in a stationary mid-range position (fig. 6). Pain or increased

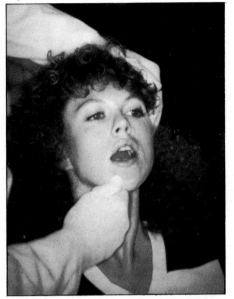

Fig. 6 Resistance test for the left lateral and medial pterygoid muscles. Pain or increased symptoms during this test are a positive sign of a muscular disorder.

symptoms during resistance testing are a positive sign of a muscular or tendon disorder.[3] It can be inferred that the source of the pain is in those muscles producing the resistance. Muscular weakness may also be appreciated, especially as it may be manifested by comparison of the lateral pterygoid muscles.

Resistance tests are an excellent method of identifying primary muscular pain, since they normally will not test positively to conditions of referred pain.[3] They are also particularly useful in assessing muscles relatively unavailable to palpation, such as the lateral pterygoids. Unfortunately, if the functional resistance tests fails to incorporate those parts of the muscles that are damaged, resistance tests may not fully disclose all primary muscle pain. Other tests (see below) are recommended to augment the impressions gained from resistance testing.

Joint and muscle loading tests
Joint clicking
Temporomandibular clicking is usually tested by stethoscope or palpation during free open and close movements. However, approximately 10% of individuals mask their clicking except when chewing a bolus of hard food. It seems justifiable to suggest that temporomandibular joint function be

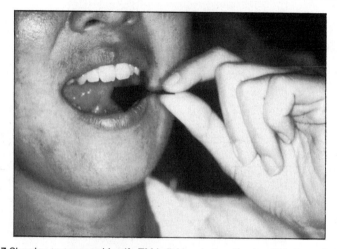

Fig. 7 Chewing test wax to identify TMJ clicking during chewing. This form of clicking is occasionally silent during free open-close jaw motion.

tested by instructing the patient to chew firm wax while the examiner lightly palpates the joints for evidence of clicking (fig. 7). This will induce clicking under dynamic functional conditions in predisposed individuals. Sometimes the click will occur only during the crossover phase of alternating bilateral chewing. This is particularly typical of hard 'knocking' that accompanies patients with advanced TMJ changes.

Traditional methods should be used to evaluate TMJ clicking outside the envelope of chewing motion. The joint may be also tested by influencing its function with lateral finger pressure over the TMJ during dynamic movements.

Joint pain

Fluoroscopy methods have demonstrated that the joint can be put under slight distraction or compression by the individual's own biting force. The bitestick (fig. 8) may be placed ipsilaterally to the symptomatic TMJ to produce joint distraction. It may be placed contralaterally to the TMJ to induce compression. These actions are most pronounced if the bitestick is placed in the second or third molar region.

If TMJ pain is due to impingement of soft tissues, ipsilateral biting will ameliorate the pain and contralateral biting will aggravate the pain (figs 8 (*a*), (*b*)). The bitestick is not specific for joint pain only, but can be diagnostic when augmented by the patient's indication that the joint is the site of provoked pain, and by the finding of tenderness by joint palpation.

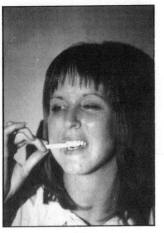
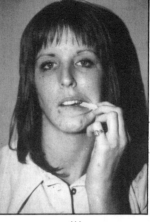

(a)   (b)

Fig. 8 Bitestick test for pain on the left side. (a) biting on the contralateral side produced left TMJ pain whereas (b) biting on the ipsilateral side gave relief. This suggested an impingement-type pain in the left TMJ; the relief with the bitestick suggested that a bite appliance might be warranted.

Muscular pain

Bitesticks, clenching, and normal functional movements may be used to provoke primary pain in the masticatory muscles. Clenching in the intercuspal position may provoke pain in both jaw openers and closers. If clenching produces pain in appropriate muscular areas, bilateral bitesticks should be tested.

Often the insertion of bilateral spacers relieves the clenching pain, suggesting to the examiner that a bite appliance may give benefit. Usually this effect will be accompanied by profound, symmetrical muscle contraction of the jaw closers.

Bitesticks may be utilised on the ipsilateral side to test elevator and lateral pterygoid muscles. The elevator muscles will be provoked by their contraction against the resistance of bitestick. If ipsilateral muscle pain is ameliorated by this test, the lateral pterygoid muscle may be involved. This muscle is slightly shortened during this test and therefore may not produce pain when biting on the stick, as compared with biting with the teeth clenched.

Symptom-provoking contacts

Muscular resistance testing can be tailored to individual mandibular

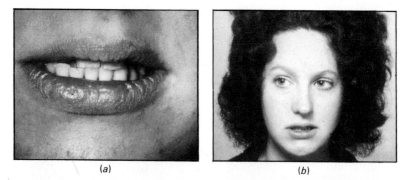

(a)   (b)

Fig. 9 (a), (b) Symptom-provoking tooth contacts. Pain produced when 'setting' selected bruxofacets together may indicate a muscular source of complaints. This directs the clinician to the type of jaw behaviour and tooth contact causing the symptoms.

behaviour. Areas of wear from bruxism or anterior tooth setting may be identified (fig. 9 (a)). The patient is instructed to set these facets in apposition with a heavy 'tooth press' for 60 seconds (fig. 9 (b)). Pain or severe fatigue provoked by this test may be identical to that reported in the chief complaint, with consequent implications as to the oral behaviour causing these complaints.[9]

Positive results from symptom-provoking tests should direct the examiner to mask the bruxofacets with a bite appliance, to alter them by selective grinding.[9] In so doing, the symptom-eliciting activity is attenuated with a concomitant reduction in muscle activity and symptoms.

Palpation

Palpation is widely accepted as a method for examining the soft and hard tissues. Among the characteristics identified are the intensity and location of tenderness, degree of muscle tonicity, trigger points, swelling, hardness and temperature, and anatomical landmarks for examination and injection.

Palpation in muscle pain diagnosis remains one of the essentials of physical examination despite the difficulty of reproducing the results.[10] The abundance of palpable tender spots in muscles has been reported in otherwise normal individuals.[4] Over-interpretation is common, owing to the normal sensitivity of some anatomical structures, the presence of inflamed nodes in the area, and hyperalgesia[11] associated with prolonged referred pain. The risk for over-reporting tenderness suggests that palpation might be used most appropriately to augment the findings of functional tests rather than as a 'stand alone' criterion for the TM disorder.[3]

Palpation of the TMJ, on the other hand, is more reliable as an indicator of joint tenderness and inflammation. Joint tenderness is not as prevalent in non-patient populations.[4] Like the muscles, the TMJ can be selectively palpated to identify localised areas of capsular tenderness, which can then be evaluated together with the results of functional bitestick tests, and other joint manipulation.

Diagnostic analgesic injections

Pain provoked by manual palpation or functional manipulation is arrested by analgesic blocking of the structure from which it emanates.[11] For this reason, it is appropriate to consider diagnostic injections for the occasional pain problem which, despite other functional testing, does not suggest a satisfactory diagnosis. Procaine or Lignocaine without adrenaline, 1% or 2%, is the recommended anaesthetic. This technique has been previously described by Bell.[12] The usual sites chosen are those typically less available for direct examination, such as the lateral pterygoid muscle.

Occasionally the TMJ is suspected as the source of earache, temporal headache, or jaw pain. Additionally, painful restriction might persuade the examiner to block the TMJ in order to better understand its source. To evaluate these problems diagnostically the auriculotemporal block[13] (described in a later paper in the series: 'Synovitis, hypomobility and deformity') is completed using the same anaesthetics described above.

In summary, physical diagnosis continues to have as its foundation an emphasis on functional tests, as contrasted with psychological findings, when diagnosing the 'TMJ case'. The implicit message from this article is that TM disorders should not be a catch-all term for any facial pain. Familiarity with the principles of diagnosis of soft tissue pain and dysfunction makes the differential diagnosis of the TM disorder more straightforward. Application of these principles to the masticatory system is recommended.

References

1 Solberg W K. Temporomandibular disorders: Background and the clinical problems. *Br Dent J* 1985; **160:** 157–161.
2 Cailliet R. *Soft tissue pain and disability.* pp 1–2. Philadelphia: F. A. Davis Co, 1977.
3 Friedman M H, Weisberg J. *Temporomandibular joint disorders, diagnosis and treatment.* pp 41–44. Chicago: Quintessence, 1985.
4 Solberg W K, Woo M S, Houston J B. Prevalence of mandibular dysfunction in young adults. *J Am Dent Assoc* 1979; **98:** 25–34.
5 Agerberg G, Österberg T. Maximal mandibular movements and symptoms of mandibular dysfunction in 70-year-old men and women. *Sven Tandlak Tidskr* 1974; **67:** 147–163.
6 Agerberg G. Maximal mandibular movements in young men and women. *Sven Tandlak Tidskr* 1974; **67:** 81–100.

7 Hansson T L, Nilner M. A study of the occurrence of symptoms of diseases of the temporomandibular joint, masticatory musculature and related structures. *J Oral Rehab* 1975; **2:** 313–325.

8 McCarty W Jr. Diagnosis and treatment of internal derangements of the articular disc and mandibular condyle. *In* Solberg W K, Clark G T (eds) *Temporomandibular joint problems: biologic diagnosis and treatment.* pp 158–160. Chicago: Quintessence, 1980.

9 Krogh-Poulsen W G, Olsson A. Management of the occlusion of the teeth. *In* Schwartz L L, Chayes C M (eds) *Facial pain and mandibular dysfunction.* pp 236–280. Philadelphia: Saunders, 1968.

10 Carlsson G E, Helkimo M, Agerberg G. Observatorsskillnader vid bettfysiologisk undersokning. *Tandlakartidningen* 1974; **66:** 565–572.

11 Bell W E. *Clinical management of temporomandibular disorders.* pp 81–98. Chicago: Year Book Medical Publishers, 1982.

12 Bell W E. *Clinical management of temporomandibular disorders.* pp 183–185. Chicago: Year Book Medical Publishers, 1982.

13 Donlon W C, Truta M P, Eversole L R. A modified auriculotemporal nerve block for regional anaesthesia of the temporomandibular joint. *J Oral Maxillofac Surg* 1984; **42:** 544–545.

5 Data collection and examination

Evaluation of mandibular function necessitates a broader surveillance of the head, neck and jaws than is generally realised. Dental examination limited to the teeth and periodontium overlooks distant problems in the muscles and joints which could be aggravated or ameliorated by dental therapy. Therefore the dentist should strive to recognise function-related symptoms in these regions so as to better predict difficulties in completing the dental task ahead. Because stress-induced muscle tension and traumatic oral habits are common causes of headache, earache, and temporomandibular problems, one must expectantly screen for these symptoms and assess their significance through examination.

The purpose of this paper is to describe an approach to effective documentation and diagnosis of signs and symptoms involving temporomandibular disorders (TMD). The task is not all that difficult. It has been shown that the majority of patients with TMD can be identified by a short questionnaire.[1] However, an abbreviated examination should be done to estimate the operative risk for precipitating clinical problems in those patients with subliminal signs.[2] Because substantial benefit accrues with conservative treatment carried out in the dental setting,[3] the evaluation and assessment of patients with suspected TMD will be emphasised.

Data collection
The usefulness of questionnaires for collecting general medical information is fully accepted. Their acknowledged purpose is to ask for information that

Table I Questionnaire for temporomandibular disorders

Yes	No	Part 1
—	—	Does your jaw make noise so that it bothers you or others?
—	—	Does your jaw get stuck so that you can't open freely?
—	—	Does it hurt when you chew or open wide to take a big bite?
—	—	Do you have earaches or pain in front of the ears?
—	—	Do you have pain in the face, cheeks, jaws, throat or temples?
—	—	Are you unable to open your mouth as far as you want to?
—	—	Do you suffer from frequent headaches?
—	—	Does your jaw 'feel tired' after a big meal or dental visit?
—	—	Are you aware of an uncomfortable bite?

Yes	No	Part 2
—	—	Are you aware that you grind your teeth at night?
—	—	Do you have a habit of clamping or 'setting' your teeth?
—	—	Do you have any jaw symptoms or headache upon waking in the morning?
—	—	Must you chew exclusively on one side?
—	—	Have you had a blow to the jaw (trauma)?
—	—	Are you a habitual gum-chewer or pipesmoker?

Yes	No	Part 3
—	—	Does the pain or discomfort disturb your sleep?
—	—	Does the pain or discomfort interfere with your daily routine or other activities?
—	—	Do you take medications or pills for pain or discomfort? (pain relievers, muscle relaxants, antidepression pills)
—	—	Does the pain or discomfort affect your appetite?
—	—	Do you find the pain or discomfort extremely frustrating or depressing?

Yes	No	Part 4
—	—	Do you suffer from arthritis or pain in other joints?
—	—	Do you suffer from nervous stomach or ulcers?
—	—	Do you suffer from constipation? colitis?
—	—	Do you suffer from back or neck pain (whiplash)?
—	—	Do you suffer from skin problems or allergies?
—	—	Have you ever been treated for a jaw muscle or jaw joint disorder?

the clinician does not want to miss, particularly if it will not be asked during the oral history. Screening for mandibular dysfunction and orofacial pain is similarly rewarding. A four-part questionnaire appears in Table I. Part 1 includes questions that identify the patient with probable TMD. Note that most of these are associated with jaw function.[1] Part 2 questions are directed to habits and other factors that may have provoked the symptoms. Part 3 documents behavioural responses in the face of symptoms. Parts 3 and 4 deal with general factors likely to be associated with a worsening prognosis. In short, patients answering positively in Parts 1 and 2 only are more likely to respond to treatment than those patients who respond to all parts of the questionnaire. The application is to not only detect symptoms, but to direct the examiner to consider the implications for prognosis.

The history should accomplish the following: (1) to identify the problem and to delve explicitly into the regional or associated symptoms; (2) to evaluate for habits, trauma and other general factors which point to the aetiology of the complaints; (3) to develop the psychosocial context (illness, suffering) accompanying the disease or disorder; (4) to identify and assess the outcome of prior treatment. The following approach may be considered.

Symptoms

The questionnaire or other information obtained prior to the visit to the surgery will alert the examiner that TM disorder should be suspected. The history should be elicited keeping in mind the key feature of TMD: painful function in the musculoskeletal tissues of the masticatory system. The pain in the area of the jaw and ear should faithfully follow deep-pain characteristics (dull aching pain punctuated by sharp or throbbing pains where severe). Primary TM pain increases with the demands of function. Resting pain without relation to function should direct the clinician to seek other causes than the muscles and TMJs.

Table II Interview checklist for TM disorders

Chief complaint	Associated functional disturbances
Mode of onset, chronicity	Altered range of jaw or neck motion
Intensity	TMJ mechanics (noise, incoordination)
Character, quality	Acute alteration of the dental occlusion
Location	
Temporal behaviour: over 24 hours; progression since onset	**Aetiology**
	Macrotrauma, overstretching of jaw
Aggravating factors: function; stress; temperature	Bruxism habit or other jaw behaviour
	Recent dental interventions
Ameliorating factors	Stress, tension, recent life events
Outcome of prior treatment	
Current medications	**Psychosocial context**
	Work
Associated pains	Relationships
Sinusache	Play
Earache	Sleep
Headache	
Neckache	
Toothache	

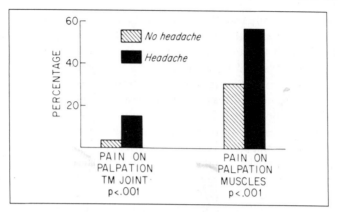

Fig. 1 Significant masticatory findings with headaches in 739 young adults.[2]

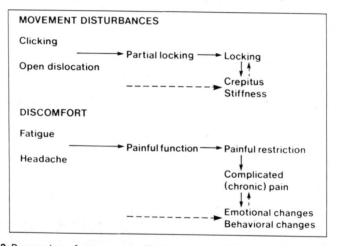

Fig. 2 Progression of temporomandibular disorders. (From Solberg W K. Current concepts on the development of TMJ dysfunction. *In* Carlson D, McNamara J A Jr and Ribbens K A (eds) *Developmental aspects of temporomandibular disorders.* pp 37–47. Ann Arbor: University of Michigan, 1985.)

The key to the elicitation of symptoms is to be explicit. Chronicity, intensity, occurrence, location, pain characteristics, aggravating and ameliorating factors and outcome of treatment should be appropriately covered (Table II). Once accomplished, a symptom review of possible associated pains is recommended; headache, neckache, toothache, sinusache and earache should be explored with relationship to the chief complaint (fig. 1).

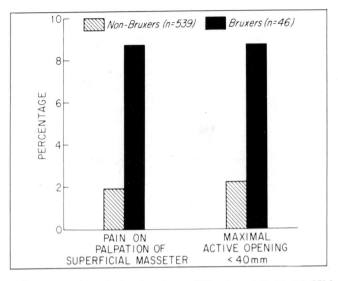

Fig. 3 Significant findings with bruxism among 739 young adults ($P < 0.05$).[2]

Look for three functional disturbances: TMJ mechanics, bite discrepancies, and range-of-motion problems (Table II). The relationship of these dysfunctions to each other and to functional pain should be documented. The sequence and progression of the symptoms should be considered (fig. 2).

Aetiology

The cause of the symptoms may be apparent as in the case of trauma or overstretching, or they may be insidious without explanation. It has been recently shown that trauma significantly characterises TMD patients when compared with an age-matched group free of TMD symptoms.[4] Bruxism and other behaviour may be active perpetuating factors (fig. 3). Emotional stress and recent life events are significant. However, extensive investigation of psychophysiological factors as causes of TM disorders resulted in the conclusion that no one particular personality trait necessarily predisposes to their development.[5] Evaluating individuals for TM disorders in terms of stress factors rather than underlying suppressed conflicts is more practical for the dentist (Table II).

Psychosocial context

It has been noted that people are more similar than varied in their response

Table III Miscellaneous symptoms possibly occurring as secondary excitatory effects via the central nervous system

Dizziness	Numbness
Fullness, ringing in the ears	Burning sensation
Facial swelling	Taste changes
Tears in eyes	Throat, eye, noise
Redness of eyes	sensitivity
Nasal congestion	Distorted vision

to illness-producing factors. This has led to the admonition, 'Every TMJ has a patient attached to it!' The implication is that the dentist is treating obscure, chronic pain and must accept, as part of his role, the obligation to render supportive psychotherapy. The dentist may be uncomfortable with this notion because dental training has been inadequate in this area.

Often, insights can be gained from the mechanics of history-taking. For example, failure of the patient to state his chief complaint clearly and concisely is diagnostic in itself. One can begin in a specific way by remembering that there are three key life events: work, relationships, and play (Table II). Review of these areas often produces insights into the patient's problem. Sleep pattern and quality are good indicators of overall functioning. Patients who wake up too early with their 'wheels already turning' often need rectification of this problem before local therapy can be successful.

It has been said that the examiner need ask the patient only one question: 'What does this problem stop you from doing?' It may be realised that the patient is avoiding social life, work, motherhood or a variety of other responsibilities behind the mask of pain and suffering.

Many of these patients are not good candidates for traditional psychiatric help; multidisciplinary approaches in a controlled setting are better solutions.

Other associated symptoms

Temporomandibular disorders have the attributes of deep pain, including secondary central excitatory effects associated with continuous deep pain input.[6] It has been hypothesised that this accounts for the complaints of ear fullness (stuffiness), ringing, altered hearing, dizziness, and other seemingly unrelated symptoms (Table III). Apart from the belief that they are centrally mediated,[6] the relationship of these symptoms to nociceptive disorders in the masticatory system is still unexplained. Feinmann and Harris[7] have pointed out the tendency of TMD to merge with other facial pain syndromes.

Table IV Tests and measures for examination

Swallowing

Range of motion
Pain-free opening
Active range of motion (AROM)
Passive range of motion (PROM)

TMJ function
Extent of movement
Free movements and chewing wax: grading of click; grading of
crepitation
Stethoscopic evaluation as needed
Diagnostic manipulation as needed

TMJ palpation for tenderness
Dorsal to joint
Lateral to joint

Resistance tests
Opening
Lateral
Protrusive

Loading tests
Unilateral bitestick: ipsilateral to symptom side; contralateral to
symptom side
Bilateral bitestick
Intercuspal clenching
Symptom-provoking contact

Muscle palpation
Masticatory group
Neck group
Neck range of motion

Neuromuscular function
Closure tests
Masseter function
Tooth contact movement
Retruded range manipulation

Occlusal analysis
Retruded position (RCP to ICP)
Zones of ICP contact
Gross occlusal interferences
Attrition and soft tissue ridging

Examination

In a previous article,[8] the principles of physical diagnosis were discussed.
Their application in examination (Table IV) will be aimed at confirming
the existence of TMD, and relating these findings to one or more of four
major diagnostic subgroups. The subgroups are: (1) acute muscular
disorders; (2) TMJ internal derangement; (3) inflammation (synovitis and

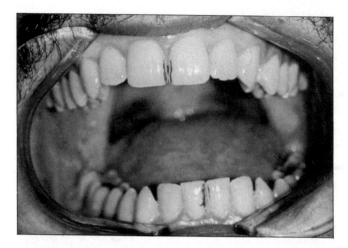

Fig. 4 Deflection of mandible and incisal point to the left. This patient had normal excursions in the horizontal plane, suggesting that the deflection was due to restriction of the ipsilateral elevator groups.

tendinitis); and (4) disorders of hypomobility and deformity. The diagnosis and management of each of these subgroups will be the topic of future papers.

Swallowing

Occasionally pharyngeal structures associated with swallowing are the source of painful function, as in the case of glossopharyngeal neuralgia or Eagle's syndrome. Testing swallowing while the jaw is biting on a tongue blade will help, if the throat is the source of the pain.

Range of motion

Testing range of motion should expose conditions of hypomobility or hypermobility and their relationship to pain and mechanical problems. A valuable first measure is maximum pain-free opening. Monitoring this measure during treatment tells much about patient progress. Active (AROM) and passive (PROM) range-of-motion tests should delineate the source of the restriction, whether articular or muscular or both.[8] If additional opening is encouraged from PROM testing, a muscular source is likely. Optimal results are obtained if the face is first sprayed with fluorimethane spray.[9] The clicking point during opening should also be indicated. Observe the trajectory of the jaw and incisal point in three planes and note deflections, deviations, and tremor (fig. 4). If opening is restricted

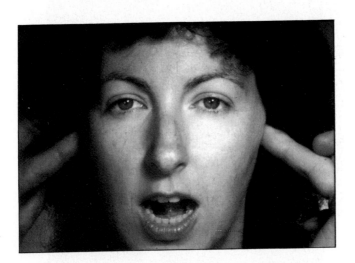

Fig. 5 Palpation of the TMJ for clicking and rough movement.

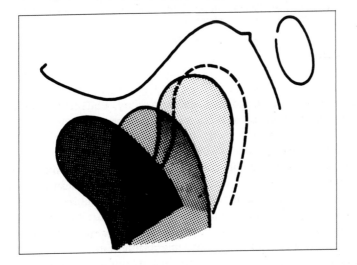

Fig. 6 Timing of the TMJ clicking should be noted according to the zones of condylar movement. Dotted line = closed position; solid line = early opening; stipple = mid-opening; dark, tone = wide open position. (From Solberg W K, Seligman D A. Temporomandibular orthopedics: A new vista in orthodontics. *In* Johnston L E (ed) *New vistas in orthodontics.* pp 148–183. Philadelphia: Lea Febiger, 1985.)

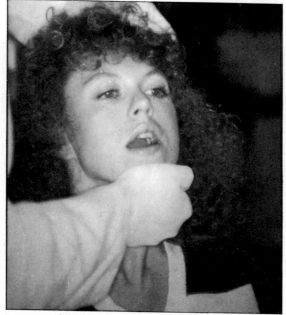

Fig. 7 Resistance test of the jaw openers. Both the lateral pterygoid muscles and the digastrics are recruited with this manoeuvre.

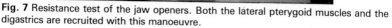

but horizontal movements are not, the restriction is more likely in the musculature.

TMJ function

Clicking is associated with disc-condyle instability, while crepitus (grating joint) indicates roughness or deterioration associated with osteoarthrosis. Multiple clicks occurring along the path of opening suggest a disc perforation or complicated changes of joint form. Reciprocal clicks (occurring both on opening and closing) are associated with anterior displacement of the articular disc, particularly so when associated with jaw shift just short of full closure. Most clicks are not troublesome. Ask the patient about any history of clicking and evaluate functional impairment. Ask if the click is becoming more troublesome. The most significant clicks are those associated with painful chewing or intermittent locking.

To test for clicking, palpate lightly over the joint capsule during free open–close movements (fig. 5). Consult the patient as to the location of the click. Judge the timing of the click according to early, intermediate, or wide open zones (respectively I, II, III) of condyle travel, and whether it occurs during opening, closing, or both (fig. 6). Note explicitly the timing and character of the click. Test the TMJs under function by making the patient chew wax.

Resistance tests

Primary muscle disorders are likely to be responsive to maximal resistance. Concomitant stimulation of noxious pain in the TMJs is avoided by doing this test without moving the joint. The procedure is as follows: with the head supported and the mouth open a finger breadth, a gradual build-up of force is generated by the hand of the examiner. The patient is instructed to resist the examiner's initiative to move the jaw. The test is interrupted if pain is produced (fig. 7). A positive response usually will include pain that mimics the pain complaint. If several muscles are involved, weigh the relative intensity of pain produced by each trial.[10]

Biting tests are another method of putting the muscles and TMJs under load (fig. 8). Because muscular resistance and biting tests may precipitate prolonged post-operative symptoms, their use during the screening of the asymptomatic patient is not recommended. Resistance testing is more useful for testing the jaw openers, while bitestick testing is more practical for testing the jaw closers.

Muscle palpation

The subjective pain pattern should be precisely diagrammed. The muscular structures are palpated using the sequence shown in figure 9. If the purpose is to screen for muscle tenderness, the bimanual approach is suggested (fig. 10). Each muscle pair is palpated simultaneously and mutually, with a slight rolling pressure of the index or middle fingers. Firm, purposeful pressure is applied, after which the examiner asks 'Do you feel any difference between the two sides?' If the answer is 'yes', ask 'Does it hurt, or is it just uncomfortable?' Tenderness may be graded as mild, moderate or severe, with severe reserved for those palpations that are associated with bodily withdrawal or eye wincing (palpebral reflex). If referred pain is suspected from the tender spot, maintain pressure up to 6 seconds, one side at a time. Ask the patient where the pain travels. These triggers can be more easily identified by palpating with the muscles under gentle stretch.

Neck range of motion is conveniently conducted at this point. The patient is asked to extend and flex the neck, and to sidebend and rotate to each side. Pain experienced during these movements should direct the examiner to consider the need for cervical evaluation in the management of this patient.

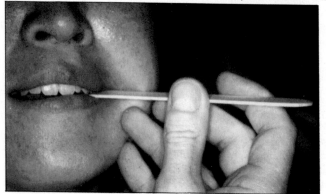

Fig. 8 Bitestick test loads the ipsilateral elevator muscles and the contralateral TMJ.

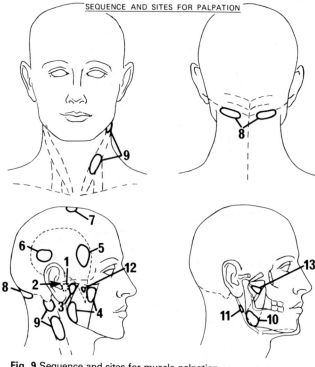

Fig. 9 Sequence and sites for muscle palpation.

Joints
(1) Lateral to capsule
(2) Dorsal to capsule (via ear)

Extra-oral musculature
(3) Deep masseter
(4) Superficial masseter
(5) Anterior temporal
(6) Posterior temporal

(7) Vertex
(8) Neck
(9) Sternocleidomastoid
(10) Medial pterygoid
(11) Posterior digastric

Intra-oral musculature
(12) Temporalis tendon
(13) Lateral pterygoid

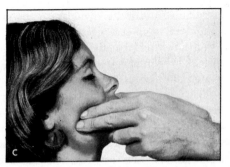

Fig. 10 Bimanual palpation of the superficial portion of the masseter muscle. (From Solberg W K. Occlusion-related pathosis and its clinical evaluation. *In* Clark J W (ed) *Clinical dentistry*. Revised edition, Volume 2, Chapter 35, 1985.)

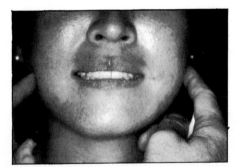

Fig. 11 Masseter function test to assess the degree and symmetry of contraction.

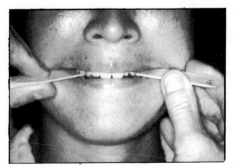

Fig. 12 Bilateral bitestick test used in conjunction with the masseter function test (cf. fig. 11).

Neuromuscular function

Under optimal mandibular function, individuals should make jaw closure to one functional end-point. This can be tested visually, then by deliberate tapping of the teeth together under stethoscopic monitoring.[11] The ability of the masseter muscles to shorten with symmetry and vigour can be tested by bimanual palpation of this muscle while directing the patient to close forcefully from light intercuspal contact (fig. 11). Asymmetrical contraction indicates occlusal instability; lack of contraction suggests muscular complications. If biting bilaterally on separators rectifies the abnormal masseter contraction, a bite appliance may be warranted (fig. 12). Guarding during rehearsed jaw excursions suggests neuromuscular splinting and associated guarding. Splinting or pain following retruded range manipulation is indicative of dysfunction in this direction of joint movement.

Occlusal analysis

Clinicians have stressed the relationship between retruded contact position (RCP) and intercuspal position. For patients having clinically stable TMJs, it seems reasonable to use RCP as a reference position from which to judge the alignment and positional requirements of occlusions in both children and adults.[12] The supporting zones of intercuspal contact should be verified

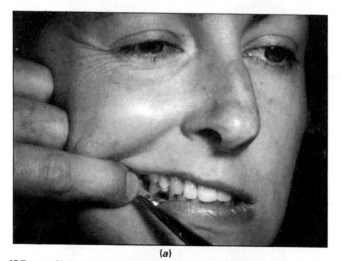

(a)

Fig. 13 Zones of intercuspal contact: (a) mylar strip held in a mosquito haemostat in order to verify contact; (b) zones of contact tested and noted on the patient's record. (I, incisor: C, canine; P, premolar; M, molar). (Same credits as in figure 6.)

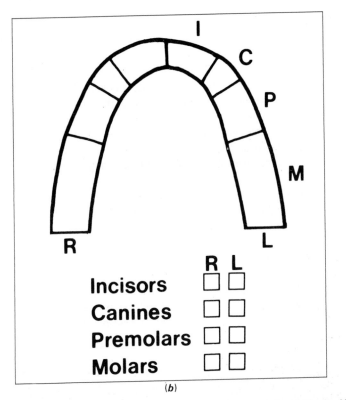

Incisors R L ☐ ☐
Canines ☐ ☐
Premolars ☐ ☐
Molars ☐ ☐

(b)

and adults.[12] The supporting zones of intercuspal contact should be verified and charted (fig. 13 (*a*)–(*b*)). The author believes this record will often be more important than dental casts registered in the articulator. Gross occlusal interferences should be noted, particularly if they are the disturbing mediotrusive (balancing) type which prevent cross-arch contact on the working inclines. Interferences incorporated in the course of dental procedures are sometimes symptom provoking.

The association of tooth wear with TMD is unclear. It appears to be more prevalent in men as opposed to women.[13] From a standpoint of dentistry, tooth wear may be a detriment to the longevity of dental restorations. Soft tissue ridging is indicative of muscle hyperactivity with or without tooth contact.

While examination procedures have been discussed with the symptomatic patient in mind, an abbreviated screening examination comprising selected tests from most of the categories is suggested. Resistance tests and bitestick tests are not recommended for screening purposes.

Conclusion

Standards of clinical practice are emerging which involve new responsibilities for the dentist in the prevention and treatment of TMD. In particular, the dentist is faced with prevalent TM findings such as clicking, jaw fatigue, and post-operative functional pains. Most of these are benign and pose no problem in practice once they are detected and dealt with by conservative measures. This paper has suggested data collection and examination approaches that have proven helpful in addressing minor or major complaints of TMD. For more information, the reader is referred to the fundamental work of Krogh-Poulsen and Olsson.[14]

References

1 Hijzen T H, Slangen J F. Myofascial pain–dysfunction: Subjective signs and symptoms. *J Prosthet Dent* 1985; **54:** 705–711.

2 Solberg W K, Woo M S, Houston J B. Prevalence of mandibular dysfunction in young adults. *J Am Dent Assoc* 1979; **98:** 25–34.

3 Mejersjö C, Carlsson G E. Long term results of treatment for temporomandibular pain and dysfunction. *J Prosthet Dent* 1983; **49:** 809–815.

4 Pullinger A G, Monteiro A A. History factors in TM disorders. (unpublished data).

5 Green C S, Olson R E, Laskin D M. Psychological factors in the etiology, progression, and treatment of MPD syndrome. *J Am Dent Assoc* 1982; **105:** 443–448.

6 Bell W E. *Orofacial pains: classification diagnosis management.* 3rd ed, pp 61–72. Chicago: Year Book Medical Publishers, 1985.

7 Feinmann C, Harris M. Psychogenic facial pain. Part I: the clinical presentation. *Br Dent J* 1984, **156:** 165–168.

8 Solberg W K. Temporomandibular disorders: physical tests in diagnosis. *Br Dent J* 1986; **160:** 273–277.

9 Travell J, Simmons D. *Myofascial pain and dysfunction: the trigger point manual,* pp 45–102. Baltimore: Williams and Wilkins, 1983.

10 Friedman M H, Weisberg J. *Temporomandibular joint disorders: diagnosis and treatment.* pp 50–54. Chicago: Quintessence, 1985.

11 Watt D M. The incidence of abnormal tooth contacts and their detection. *In* Anderson D J, Matthews B (eds) *Mastication.* p. 242. Bristol: Wright, 1976.

12 Solberg W K. Current concepts on the development of TMJ dysfunction. *In* Carlson D, McNamara J A Jr, Ribbens K A (eds) *Developmental aspects of temporomandibular disorders.* pp 37–47. Ann Arbor: University of Michigan, 1985.

13 Droukas B, Lindee C, Carlsson G E. Occlusion and mandibular dysfunction: a clinical study of patients referred for functional disturbances of the masticatory system. *J Prosthet Dent* 1985; **53:** 402–406.

14 Krogh-Poulsen W G, Olsson A. Management of the occlusion of the teeth. *In* Schwartz L, Chayes C M (eds) *Facial pain and mandibular dysfunction.* pp 236–280. Philadelphia: W B Saunders, 1968.

6 Masticatory myalgia and its management

Of the signs associated with temporomandibular disorders (TMD), muscle tenderness is the most prominent finding (fig. 1). Jaw incoordination and restriction are sometimes concomitants of muscle pain, and it is important to identify whether they relate to muscular or joint conditions. Muscular disorders may appear independent of TMJ arthropathy but usually not vice versa. Several distinct muscular problems can be identified. They tend to form a continuum ranging from subliminal tension and deficiency to disabling pain and restriction. As a result, the diagnostic subgroups tend to become blurred in the clinical setting. Nevertheless, one should delineate the various muscular subgroups because their treatment is not always the same. This paper describes clinical subgroups associated with myalgia and reviews methods useful to their management by the dentist. Since muscular pain is a major aspect of TMD, the proposed methods may also be recognised as the essentials of initial conservative management for most forms of TMD.

Pain of muscular origin

One of the causes of myalgia in the chewing muscles is stress-induced hyperactivity built up through oral habits and other self-destructive behaviour.[1] An equally tenable source of muscle pain is local functional hyperactivity in the form of postural guarding and functional overload secondary to structural abnormalities.[2] Yemm[3] has proposed a combined role of these two factors. Clinical recognition of these phenomena may be first associated with fatigue, tremor and neuromuscular deficiency, followed in time by alterations which take on a more organic character.

During prolonged anxiety and tension, the pain threshold for a standard sustained contraction is reduced.[4] Once jaw muscle tightness has reached a sufficiently high level, the stage is set for the first attack of jaw pain. Frequently, the event that precipitates the clinical pain is a traumatic one: a sudden unaccustomed chewing behaviour or overstretching the jaw muscles during a dental visit. General perpetuating factors are nutritional inadequacy, endocrine disorders, and viral infections.[5] Muscle pain may be self-sustaining owing to reflex contraction of the muscle. Some individuals acquire coping behaviour that results in the recruitment of distant muscle groups to perform simple tasks. This explains why neck and throat symptoms are seen in association with TMD and sometimes are ameliorated by stomatognathic treatments. One should also look for the multi-muscle syndromes (fibrositis) that are characterised by generalised body aches and pains.[6]

Muscular disorders
Muscular disorders involve not only the muscles themselves but also the investing fascia which carry major nerves and vessels serving to provide nutrition, defence and repair. The pain, therefore, may arise from a combination of tissues. This has been recognised by using the term myofascial pain and dysfunction.[7]

Early signs
The earliest muscular disorders have a 'neuromuscular' character.

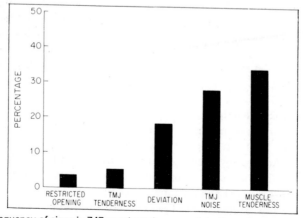

Fig. 1 Frequency of signs in 747 unselected young adults (from Solberg W K, Woo M W, Houston J B. Prevalence of mandibular dysfunction in young adults. *J Am Dent Assoc* 1979; **98**: 25–34).

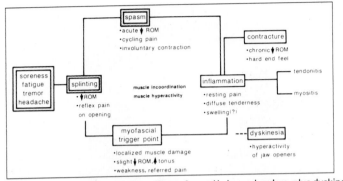

Fig. 2 Subgroups of muscular disorders. Those framed in heavy borders, plus dyskinesia, are more neuromuscular in character. The remaining subgroups are more organic in character.

Soreness, fatigue, and headache are common subjective symptoms. Weakness and tremor in the jaw openers are objective symptoms (fig. 2). Muscle splinting is characterised by these symptoms plus mild functional pain, particularly in opening and chewing. A key feature is functional limitation, which is neutralised by spray-stretch therapy.[7] Muscle splinting occurs in response to the presence of muscle or joint injury, or secondary to bruxism. Protracted splinting may include muscle spasm.[5]

Spasm

Acute spasm involves sudden involuntary muscle contracture that is maintained over time (fig. 2). The muscle is shortened, which causes pain when the muscle is stretched. Lateral pterygoid muscle involvement leads to disruption in the occlusion of the teeth (figs 3 (*a*)–(*b*)). Individuals with forceful clenching and tension are at special risk. Spasm may be secondary to continuous deep pain input from other sites.[8] As such, its exuberance may mask other problems. Diagnostic analgesic blocks made in the spastic muscle will relieve the pain and allow therapeutic stretching. Post-operative trismus may occur following surgical procedures or mandibular block injection. When prolonged, trismus may be interrupted by inject-stretch techniques. Hysterical trismus is soft tissue restriction that is a sequela of ongoing emotional conflict. It is rare in the author's experience.

Myofascial pain

Myofascial pain arises from a trigger point (TP) in a muscle and its associated fascia. According to Simons,[5] the trigger point is a hyperirritable spot that refers pain in a predictable pattern. If the TP causes referred pain

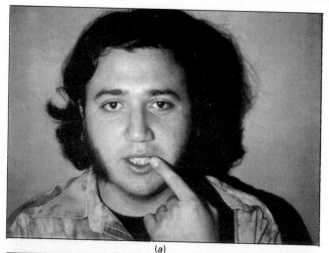

(a)

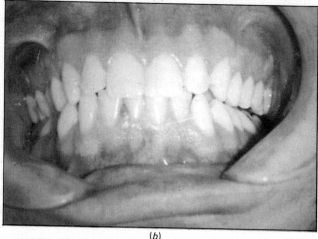

(b)

Fig. 3 Patient with acute spasm of the left lateral pterygoid muscle: (a) awareness of bite discrepancy; (b) muscle spasm causes jaw shift to the contralateral side.

during activity, or worse, at rest, it is termed 'active'. 'Latent' TPs are tender spots that may refer pain when provoked by the examiner. Often, the TP is located in a non-symptomatic muscle. Deep referred pain, with or without muscle shortening, is characteristically observed (fig. 2).

Clinically, myofascial TPs begin (and may resolve) as a neuromuscular dysfunction, but progress to a dystrophic phase at an unpredictable pace. The TP causes shortening of a taut band of associated muscle fibres that weakens and restricts full lengthening of the muscle. Therefore some active

TPs will cause pain during movement that either stretches or forcefully loads the muscle.[5] Active TPs often are accompanied by facial swelling, lacrimation, and associated muscle spasm.[5] Diagnostic blocks will completely remove the pain if made at the TP, but will give equivocal results when only the area of referred pain is injected. Unrelenting myofascial pain and dysfunction can progress to muscle inflammation (myositis, fibromyositis).

Myositis

The myositic muscle is tender, sometimes perceptibly swollen, and is irritated by almost any functional demand. Management of myositis is difficult and is usually not benefited by treatments that abate myospasm. For example, myositis is irritated by analgesic injection. The results of bite appliance therapy are equivocal. Recognition of the problem often occurs after frustrating attempts to quell the pain. The most appropriate strategy is to prescribe anti-inflammatory drugs, even resorting to short-term oral prednisone in severe cases.[7] A completely soft diet and other minimal demand on jaw use is important. Rest, coupled with gentle motion, is recommended (fig. 2).

Dyskinesia

Orofacial dyskinesia is recognised by imprecise and erratic mandibular movement. This proprioceptive problem is usually evident during excursive movements. In severe cases, some individuals suffer from the inability to bring their teeth together. There seems to be a reflex inhibition of the jaw closers by the digastric and lateral pterygoid muscles. Pronounced dyskinesia is rare, and is seen in older individuals with malocclusions that are in various states of disrepair. These difficult cases are approached by first using a thick bite appliance, which then is gradually reduced to normal vertical dimension. Adjunctive neuromuscular training is helpful (fig. 2).

Initial therapy

The most important and universal treatment for controlling muscular disorders, or any TMD, is counselling and explanation. Ironically, it is the lack of explanation on the part of doctors that is often the source of patient complaints. For example, in a study by Packard,[9] headache patients rated explanation as more desirable than medication (Table I). Giving the patient the attention and concern he really needs is enough to produce the placebo effect. The foundation of this approach lies in comprehensive diagnosis and

Table I Primary concern over headache: opinion of physicians and self-report of the patient (%)[9]

Physicians (n = 50)		Patients (n = 91)
96	—————pain relief—————	69
68	—————explanation—————	77
68	—————medication—————	20

the ability to anticipate outcome with or without specific therapy.[10] Acknowledgement of the problem with assurance that most patients get well in three to four months with conservative treatment is fundamental.[11]

Appropriate explanation for TMD comprises two general objectives as advocated by Bell.[12] The first principle is to control the pain. The goal is not to abolish all pain, since this would only encourage injudicious use of the injured part. Therefore, pain-killing narcotic analgesics are counter-productive. Functional pain serves to remind the patient to avoid that activity and initiates specific behaviour that will allow traumatised tissues to recover.[12] Non-addictive analgesics or non-steroidal anti-inflammatory drugs are useful to battle continuous pain. Diazepam is warranted as a short-term therapy when anxiety and muscle spasm are predominant. Often overlooked are effective thermal measures for producing regional analgesia (moist heat) and anaesthesia (ice). Thermal measures (see below), particularly moist heat, promote relaxation and resolution of tissue damage.

An equally effective general objective is to minimise functional demands. Rest with gentle motion, mechanically soft diet taken in small morsels, and avoidance of wide opening are the means by which this is accomplished. If the examiner suspects inflammation of the muscle or tendons, an all-liquid diet for 7–10 days or more is advised. Axis-opening exercises originating from the resting jaw position are helpful (see below).

Specific therapy

Aetiology

The most important objective is to identify and eliminate the cause: if it is traumatic muscle injury, promote rest and resolution; if it is forceful clenching, deal with forceful closing behaviour; if it is tension, prescribe graded relaxation and counselling; if it is alignment of the jaws or mandibular instability, institute measures to rectify same. When appropriate, time should be taken to discuss the role of emotional stress in creating muscle tension in the gnathic system (fig. 4). In so doing, the

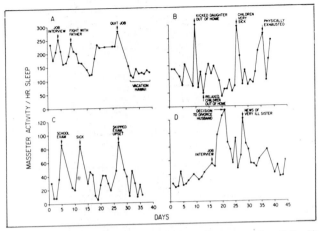

Fig. 4 Results of portable electronic measures of masticatory muscle activity. Nocturnal electromyographic levels of four females with bruxism recorded under normal activities and environment. For example, subject A experienced a dramatic drop in bruxism during her vacation in Hawaii. (From Rugh J D, Solberg W K. Electromyographic studies of bruxist behaviour, before and during treatment. *Calif Dent Assoc* 1975; **3**: 56-59.)

dentist demonstrates that healing and health maintenance are dependent upon the patient's input and willingness to actively participate in the therapy.

Physical measures

Either heat or cold relieves muscle soreness, but moist heat is perhaps the easiest to apply in the home. Cold, in the form of ice or Fluori-Methane

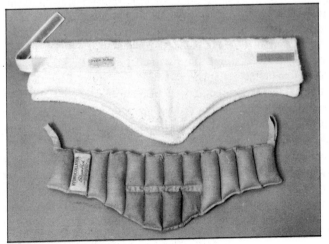

(a)

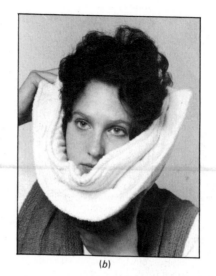

(b)

Fig. 5 (a) Moist heat pack and sleeve available commercially; (b) Proper application of moist heat pack. Heat is always applied to both sides of the face.

spray, is usually better for immediate use against muscle spasm. The advantage of moist heat is that steam is brought into contact with the skin, presumably with a greater stimulus to circulation. It is an effective tissue preparation for stretching, mobilisation or massage. Alternate application of two hot towels or the use of commercial heat-retaining packs accomplishes this purpose (figs 5 (a)–(b)). Heat is applied bilaterally, regardless of the site of pain. It is applied for 20 minutes, three times a day or more as feasible. Avoid burning the skin. Analgesia is obtained only during application. Many physical therapies such as heat, cold, medications, electrical stimulation, acupuncture, and vapocoolant sprays, have a beneficial effect on abnormal muscular tissues. Even though these modalities soothe the injured part, they do not restore physiological status and therefore are not recommended as sole measures in treatment. Therapeutic motion (mobilisation) is the key to restoring and perpetuating musculoskeletal function.

In the dental setting, the spray-stretch technique is an effective method for preparation of the muscles prior to mobilisation (fig. 6). Fluori-Methane is sprayed on the skin over previously identified TPs, resulting in momentary desensitisation of the muscle. During this period, the jaws are passively stretched to gain increased opening. The examiner should be knowledgeable in the technique before using it on patients.[7] The technique is based on the rationale that muscles brought to their physiological resting length will cease to be painful. Treatment is continued at home by the application of moist heat followed by gentle stretching. If results are obtained, spray-stretch is continued every other day until range of motion is normal and the pain is gone. Failure of this procedure should direct the

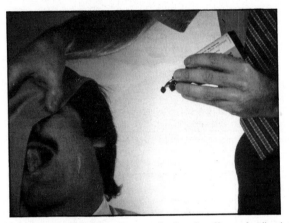

Fig. 6 Fluori-Methane spray is used to temporarily alter the afferent feedback of muscle trigger points, while the muscles are under gentle stretch. Passive stretch follows application of Fluori-Methane spray.

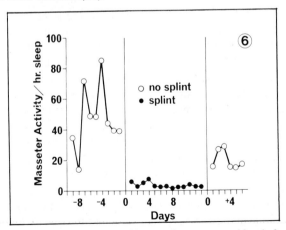

Fig. 7 Cumulative nightly electromyographic recordings on one subject before, during, and after short term splint therapy. Nocturnal masseteric muscle activity, as measured by electromyography, was reduced immediately following the insertion of a full arch maxillary stabilisation splint.[15]

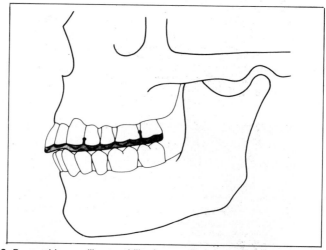

Fig. 8 Removable maxillary stabilisation appliance used for masticatory muscle disorders.

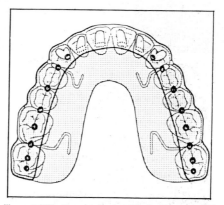

Fig. 9 Full arch maxillary stabilisation appliance. Occlusal contact scheme: black marks, intercuspal position contact scheme made by the canine and posterior functional cusps; white marks, excursive guidance involving principally the anterior teeth.

clinician to consider other diagnoses, for example muscular contracture, capsular fibrosis, or TMJ synovitis.

Muscular disorders are manifested by incoordinated and excessive condylar protrusion during jaw movements. Therefore, prescribed retraining exercises should accompany the regimen of spray-stretch/home therapy. These fall in the category of neuromuscular retraining. The axis-opening exercise is a method for retraining or relearning mandibular movements.[13] This exercise involves making symmetrical opening and closing movements with the jaw in a centred hinge position. Increased strengthening of painful muscles tends to aggravate the condition.[7] With gradual recovery, however, the muscles may be exercised under light to moderate loads (resistance exercises).

Bite appliances

Myalgia is the symptom that has the best experimental evidence to support bite appliances as a highly effective treatment.[14] These results probably occur owing to an alteration in the patient's muscle activity patterns. Bite appliances are less likely to be effective on patients with severe symptoms.[14] Their usefulness in neutralising the effects of bruxism (attrition, muscle fatigue) has been supported by investigative studies (fig. 7).[15,16] In particular, the most valid evidence regarding splint effectiveness has been documented on the full arch stabilisation splint (fig. 8).[14]

Table II Stabilisation splint criteria

Occlusal criteria
(1) Appliance stable on teeth;
(2) RCP[a] and MCP[b] contact distribution: multipointed, widely distributed contacts;
(3) MCP stability: Posterior vertical stops; incisor teeth in slight infra-contact;
(4) RCP-MCP relationship: RCP and MCP in the same sagittal plane; MCP and RCP are nearly identical;
(5) Smooth gliding contact in all excursions (incisal and/or canine disclusion optional);
(6) MCP: precise and repeatable.

Technique for verification of criteria
(1) Stability—no hint of movement to tipping forces;
(2) RCP-MCP distribution—RCP: red inked ribbon on dry surface; MCP: blue inked marking paper;
(3) Vertical stops—Mylar strips held firmly by asking subject 'close on your back teeth, both sides at the same time'; mylar strip slips through incisal contact region;
(4) RCP-MCP: Observe no slide from RCP to MCP;
(5) Guidance: Use full-arch red-blue paper. Mark excursion in red, then vertical stops in blue;
(6) MCP: 'solid' MCP tapping by patient in upright position; patient verifies 'even' contact.

---

[a] Retruded contact position on splint
[b] Muscular contact position on splint

The main aim of a stabilisation splint is to create one functional end-point of closure compatible with joint and muscle harmony. Splints are particularly useful in muscular disorder patients in whom immediate establishment of optimal occlusal relations is hampered by tipped or missing teeth, cross-bite, infra-occlusion, or in patients where 'diagnosis by treatment' trial is necessary.

There should be no uncontrolled tooth movement caused by appliance use. Appliances should be stable, retentive, and placed on the arch that is least intact. There should be no deflection from a reflex closure. Appliances should be adjusted at intervals until stability is clinically obvious. Criteria for insertion and balancing the appliance are summarised in Table II. The recommended occlusal contact scheme is shown in Figure 9.

The appliance is placed and carefully adjusted according to the criteria in Table II (see also figs 10 (*a*)–(*b*)). Generally the patient is instructed to

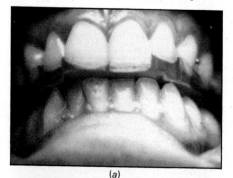

(*a*)

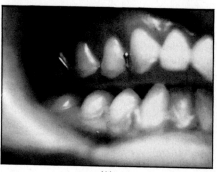

(*b*)

Fig. 10 Maxillary stabilisation appliance. (*a*) Contact relationship of the lower anterior teeth in the intercuspal position. The incisors are slightly out of contact. The canines are in full contact. (*b*) The canines and posterior teeth are in full contact in the intercuspal position.

wear the splint constantly, day and night. If the patient has pain during chewing, the splint should be worn during meals. As treatment progresses, an evaluation of the occlusal relationship to the splint will reveal discrepancies from minor jaw shift. Judgement should be exercised in determining: (1) whether definitive occlusal adjustment is advisable, (2) whether the splint should be worn indefinitely, nights only, or (3) whether the splint treatment therapy should be discontinued without making occlusal changes. Both occlusal adjustment (coronoplasty) and splint therapy can reduce some forms of headache and other forms of TMD. However, it has been shown that counselling, neuromuscular training, and bite appliances are more effective, especially in reducing the clinical signs of dysfunction.[17] Occlusal adjustment without prior splint therapy is performed when an obvious connection can be made between the symptoms and recent occlusal changes. If initial adjustment is made, the patient should be advised of the possibility that a bite appliance may be necessary later.

Trial by discontinuing the appliance that was associated with symptom relief is often a reliable method of determining whether the post-appliance occlusion needs definitive adjustment. The muscular disturbance may be the result of transient traumatic conditions rather than continuous parafunction. Therefore occlusal therapy is not mandatory following splint therapy unless clear cut occlusal loading problems from an interference or habitual bruxism are evident. The evident multifactorial causes for TM pain and dysfunction argue against dogmatic treatment methods.

Conclusions

Myalgia constitutes a major category of TMD, and it is one that can be successfully treated in the general dental setting by relatively straightforward procedures. Efforts should be made to identify the type of muscular problem before treatment starts, because they are not all treated alike.

Methods discussed in this article are also applicable as general measures for other forms of TMD. Indeed, myalgia often appears in combination with arthralgia and TMJ dysfunction. The suggested behavioural, physical and orthopaedic modalities, conducted in an atmosphere of supportive psychotherapy and informed consent, are likely to result in favourable patient response.

References

1 Solberg W K, Clark G T, Rugh J D. Nocturnal electromyographic evaluation of bruxism patients undergoing short term splint therapy. *J Oral Rehab* 1975; **2**: 215–223.
2 Møller E. The myogenic factor in headache and facial pain. *In* Kawamura Y, Dubner, R (eds) *Oral-facial sensory and motor function*, pp 225–239. Tokyo: Quintessence, 1981.
3 Yemm R. A neurophysiological approach to the pathology and aetiology of temporomandibular dysfunction. *J Oral Rehab* 1985; **12**: 343–353.
4 Dorpat T L. Mechanisms of muscle pain. Thesis, Seattle: University of Washington, 1982.
5 Simons D G. Myofascial pain syndrome due to trigger points: 1. Principles, diagnosis and perpetuating factors. *Manual Medicine* 1985; **1**: 67–71.
6 Simons D G. Myofascial pain syndromes due to trigger points: 2. Treatment and single-muscle syndromes. *Manual Medicine* 1985; **1**: 72–77.
7 Travell J G, Simons D G. *Myofascial pain and dysfunction: trigger point manual*, pp 45–102. Baltimore: Williams and Wilkins, 1983.
8 Bell W B. *Clinical management of temporomandibular disorder*, pp 81–95. London: Year Book Medical, 1982.
9 Packard R C. What does the headache patient want? *Headache* 1979; **19**: 370–374.
10 Solberg W K. Temporomandibular disorders: Background and the Clinical Problems. *Br Dent J* 1986; **160**: 157–162.
11 Nel H. Myofascial pain-dysfunction syndrome. *J Prosthet Dent* 1978; **40**: 438–441.
12 Bell W B. *Clinical management of temporomandibular disorders*, pp 190–213. Chicago: Year Book Medical, 1982.
13 Yavelow I, Forster I, Winiger M. Mandibular relearning. *Oral Surg* 1973; **36**: 632–641.
14 Clark G T. Occlusal therapy: occlusal appliances. *In* Laskin D, Greenfield W, Gale E *et al.* (eds). *The president's conference on the examination, diagnosis, and management of temporomandibular disorders*, pp 137–146. Chicago: American Dental Association, 1983.
15 Solberg W K, Clark G T, Rugh J D. Nocturnal electromyographic evaluation of bruxism patients undergoing short term splint therapy. *J Oral Rehab* 1975; **2**: 215–223.
16 Clark G T, Beemsterboer P L, Solberg W K, Rugh J D. Nocturnal electromyographic evaluation of myofascial pain dysfunction in patients undergoing occlusal splint therapy. *J Am Dent Assoc* 1979; **99**: 607–611.
17 Wenneberg B, Nyström T, Carlsson G E. Occlusal equilibration and other stomatognathic treatment in patients with mandibular dysfunction and headache. Manuscript. Gothenberg: Department of Stomatognathic Physiology, Faculty of Dentistry, November 1985.

Hydrocollator Steam Pack: Chattanooga Pharmacol Co., Chattanooga, Tennessee 37045, USA.
Fluori-Methane Spray: Gebauer Chemical Co., Cleveland, Ohio 441104, USA.

---

7 Management of internal derangement

Internal derangement is an orthopaedic term encompassing a variety of disorders that have one thing in common: they cause mechanical disturbances and impediments to joint function. A deluge of new information has established internal derangement as a major subgroup of temporomandibular disorders.[1,2] In the temporomandibular joints (TMJs), this condition includes displacement and deformation of the articular disc in addition to considerations of altered condyle position, remodelling, and joint hypermobility. The signs of TMJ derangement (TMJD) are clicking, dysfunctional condylar motion, and/or locking. While derangement originates as a mechanical interference, the most important clinical symptom is capsular pain during function, leading to muscular pain and unilateral temporal headaches.

Patients with troublesome TMJD exhibit a characteristic clinical picture that is progressive and disabling. However, if the structural mechanisms of TMJD are appreciated by the dentist, many TMJD patients who previously would have been categorised as 'functional' and therefore given stress-reduction counselling might be more appropriately treated within an orthopaedic framework. The theme of this paper is one of selected approaches to the diagnosis and treatment of TMJD as it unavoidably presents in the dental setting.

Characteristic features
A well-known feature of TMJD is anteromedial displacement of the articular disc. Rarely, the displacement is in the posterior direction.[3]

Although this problem was described many years ago,[4,5] it was not until 1978 that the mechanism was convincingly documented by arthrotomography.[6] Autopsy findings and arthrography have demonstrated marked changes in disc position (figs 1 (*a*)–(*b*)) plus distortion and folding of the disc at terminal mouth opening. The above changes have been reaffirmed by subsequent arthrographic[7] and surgical[8] studies.

Temporomandibular internal derangement involves three clinical stages of severity: painless clicking, acute locking, and painful function. Stage one involves painless TMJ clicking, brought about by the anteriorly positioned disc resuming a correct relationship with the condyle (fig. 2). The clicking sound is caused by the impact of the disc-condyle complex against the articular eminence.[9] Stage one TMJD also may be marked by the debut of open condyle dislocation, followed by chronic clicking. Open dislocation is likely to involve complete over-ride of the anterior band of the articular disc by the condyle.

Clicking is usually reciprocal, a condition that is recognised because the click occurs at a point of more condylar translation than the closing click. In reciprocal clicking, the opening click is louder than the closing click because, on opening, the condyle snaps over the disc's posterior band, impacting against the dense central part of the articular disc (fig. 2).[9] Stage one TMJD may be insignificant and stationary, or it may become a painful experience. It is not uncommon for benign stage one TMJD to persist for 5 to 10 years before stage two is precipitated by some factor such as trauma, sudden unusual movement, or excessive stretching.

Stage two TMJD is characterised by persistent displacement of the

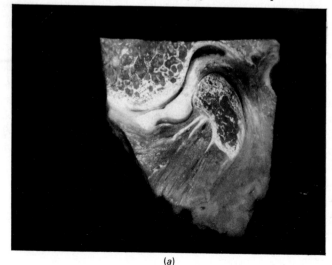

(a)

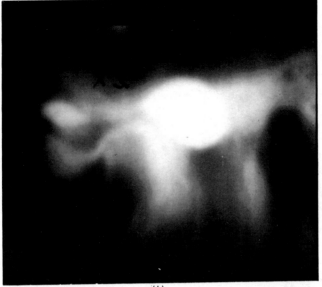

(b)

Fig. 1 (a) Sagittal cut through the medial aspect of a human temporomandibular joint from a 33-year-old female with an excellent dentition. The articular disc is totally displaced and exhibits marked distortion in shape. (b) TMJ arthrotomogram of 28-year-old female with TMJD. Projection taken with the jaw at maximal opening (anterior to the left). Displacement and distortion of the articular disc resemble the findings of the autopsy specimen in (a).

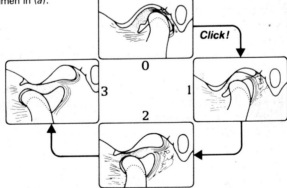

Fig. 2 The clicking TMJ. A drawing of a prolapsed articular disc (view 0). Reduction of the prolapsed disc occurs during opening (views 0 and 1). The disc is in a stable position during movement from views 1 to 3.

The clicking sound is produced as the condyle bumps over the thickened posterior border of the articular disc (from Solberg W K, Seligman D A. Temporomandibular orthopedics: a new vista in orthodontics. *In* Johnson L E (ed) *New vistas in orthodontics.* pp 148–183. Philadelphia: Lea and Febiger, 1985).

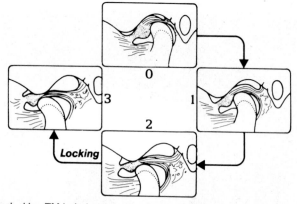

Fig. 3 The locking TMJ. A drawing of persistent anterior displacement of the articular disc without reduction in all phases of mouth opening (views 0–3). This condition usually follows periods of clicking and may progress to painful jamming of the disc (same credits as in fig. 2).

articular disc, known as locking, because it arrests condyle motion at mid-opening (fig. 3). Individuals experiencing locking first become adept at unlocking their jaw only to appear at the dentist when the locking becomes unmanageable. The complaint is usually one of restriction rather than pain. Nevertheless, acute stage two locking deserves immediate attention. Purposeful TMJ manipulation and stabilisation of the jaw are indicated rather than one limited to a course of rest and physiotherapy that is appropriate for acute muscular problems (see below).

Stage three TMJD involves a continuation of the persistent disc displacement through all phases of jaw function (fig. 3). Despite this, there is progressively less restriction of opening over time but often with increasing functional pain and disability. The disc gradually becomes distorted and folded on opening, often causing exquisite pain over a prolonged period of time (figs 4 (*a*)–(*b*)). Painful function due to inflammation becomes the paramount problem as the symptoms merge with clinical signs of osteoarthritis.[1] Unresolved late stage TMJD patients are therefore characterised by chronic arthralgia, synovitis, joint restriction and adhesions. Ironically, radiographs are frequently normal in the chronic locking patient and therefore diagnosis is dependent on informed clinical observation and TMJ arthrography.

In summary, TMJD consists of three clinical stages which vary greatly in progressivity and severity. Indeed, there is evidence that TMJD symptoms resolve following a clinical course of from three to five years.[10] Moreover, all stages of TMJD may be silent or self-limiting, thus giving the patient little motivation for seeking treatment.

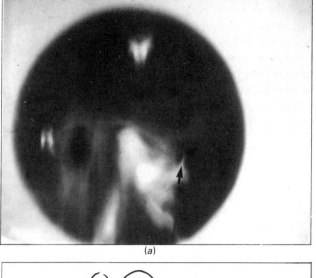

(a)

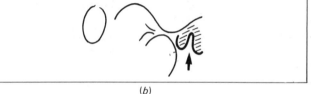

(b)

Fig. 4 (a) Arthrotomogram of a folded articular disc at full opening. Arrow indicates inferior aspect of the folded disc. (b) Diagram of the findings seen in (a). Folded disc is depicted with hatched lines.

Diagnosis

Pattern recognition is a key to the diagnosis of TMJD, as in most forms of patient evaluation. Clinical data suggest that women in their twenties and early thirties are more prone to develop troublesome TMJD than men.[1] When confronted with the patient complaining of temporomandibular pain–dysfunction, the examiner should expectantly inquire about the progressive stages of TMJD: clicking, locking, painful limitation. The aim is to identify data that point to one specific stage, because each stage is managed differently. Remember the fundamental rule: the locking joint does not click and the clicking joint does not lock.[11] The examiner should be open to the possibility of TMJD occurring secondarily in response to some form of constriction in the opposite joint. The silent TMJ may be the more involved of the two, with neither the patient nor the dentist aware of structural changes in the TMJs.

Despite the attention placed by the patient on pain, look for three important dysfunctional signs characteristic of TMJD: TMJ noise, molar bite discrepancy, and sudden restriction (locking) emanating from the TMJ area. Often these prior events will be forgotten by the patient, whose pain is demanding their full attention. For example, in one study,[12] all TMJD patients demonstrated interferences on the ipsilateral side. This finding is probably the result of disc displacement producing a reduced joint space and consequent reduced vertical dimension on the symptomatic side.[12] In

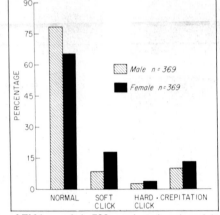

Fig. 5 Prevalence of TMJ sounds in 738 unselected young adults. More women than men were found to exhibit clicking ($P<0\cdot01$).[14]

short, pointedly assess the patient for specific dysfunctions associated with TM disorders because this information may be crucial to treatment planning.

Unilateral headache, retro-orbital pain, and pain in the supporting musculature are frequently associated with stage three TMJD. The muscular response has been studied and is interpreted as an arthrokinetic reflex caused by distraction.[12] Bruxism, especially the nocturnal type, requires detection and management. In stage three, mechanical problems tend to lessen over time, allowing more range of movement. Consequently, some patients with chronic TMJD appear almost as if they have normal joint mechanics. This clinical picture mimics myofascial pain–dysfunction, increasing the risk for misdiagnosis.

Clicking
Clicking occurs in 20 to 30% of individuals over the age of 15 years.[13,14] Young women have greater prevalence of clicking than men (fig. 5).[13,14] In

view of the widespread occurrence of clicking, its management requires careful judgement. The majority of individuals who are aware of TMJ

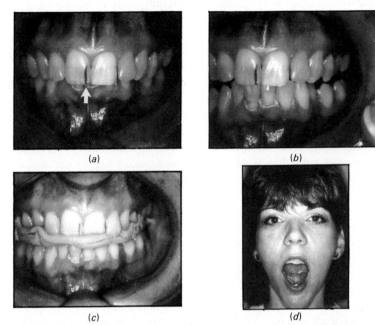

(a)   (b)

(c)   (d)

Fig. 6 The right TMJ is tested to determine whether TMJ clicking can be arrested. (a) Mid-line landmarks identified at the intercuspal position. (b) After opening beyond the clicking point, the patient closes in a slight protrusive relationship without triggering the click. (c) Softened hard-type index reproduces the position in (b). Note slight over-correction to the contralateral side (compare mid-lines). (d) Opening and closing verify that the click has been predictably arrested.

clicking are not bothered much by them; many clicking symptoms can be dealt with by explanation and education as to preventive measures.

Pronounced clicking and pain during chewing are the most problematical, but this occurs in a minority of clicking patients. Clicking during chewing occurs near the intercuspal position. These clicks can be stabilised by unconventional forward repositioning of the mandible, known as repositioning therapy (see below). Clicks occurring in other zones of the condyle path or greater than 20-mm mouth opening are not likely to respond to specific TMJ repositioning. Repositioning therapy to arrest bilateral TMJ clicking shares an equally poor prognosis. The medial direction of the disc displacement on each side makes stabilisation of both discs along a sagittal plane highly problematical.

Treatment of the painless click is generally unwarranted owing to the lack of predictability that this symptom will generate future problems. However, treatment of the painless click is potentially justified if the noisy joint becomes a social embarrassment to the patient. Overall, successful outcome of TMJD management should not depend upon the elimination of the click. Therefore, adequate orientation of the patient on the goals of therapy is important.

If the complaints of the patient suggest that stabilisation of the click might be appropriate, the joint should be tested to see if the click can be stopped in a definitive way. To do this, identify the mid-line landmarks at the intercuspal position (fig. 6(*a*)). Ask the patient to open beyond the clicking point. Then instruct the patient to close along a protruded symmetrical path that is visually referenced according to the mid-line landmarks. Closure should terminate in a slight protrusive relationship just short of the clicking point. Note that the jaw mid-line is initially over-corrected about 1 mm to the contralateral side (fig. 6(*b*)). This slight asymmetrical forward movement positions the condyle in a slight anteromedial direction, more directly centred under the usual location of the displaced disc.

When the patient has learned this manoeuvre, place four thicknesses of slightly softened hard-type wax over the maxillary teeth and repeat the previous exercise. On closure from the open protruded position, the teeth should engage the wax just prior to the clicking point, terminating in a slight protrusive relationship. This will usually produce a wax index that moves the mandible from 1 to 2 mm forward and open in roughly equal amounts (fig. 6(*c*)). Next, remove, chill, and replace the wax index. Use denture adhesive on the palatal side of the wax for retention. Observe the patient on opening and closing to verify that the click is arrested and that the patient is comfortable with the resultant maxillomandibular relationship (fig. 6(*d*)). If the decision is made to provide a bite appliance to reposition the mandible, the index is used to relate the dental casts during its fabrication.

Management of TMJD
Repositioning appliance
The correction of altered condyle position in patients with TM disorders has been advocated for many years.[15,16] However, this approach is not widely accepted because it is now known that condyle position is variable, even in asymptomatic individuals. Nevertheless, repositioning of the mandible for specific stages of TMJD has become more accepted because

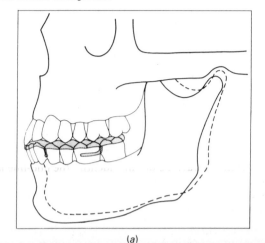

(a)

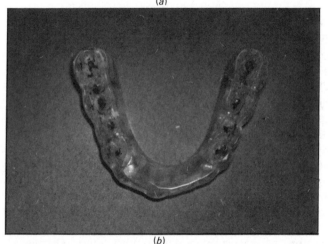

(b)

Fig. 7 (a) Mandibular repositioning appliance slightly advancing the mandible from a concentric condylar position. (b) Occlusal view of mandibular repositioning appliance revealing deep fossas which act to guide the mandible to the advanced position.

of its clinical success in normalising symptoms, particularly clicking.[17,18] With the aid of TMJ radiographs, the positioning is either made to a concentric condyle position or to an over-corrected anterior position, depending upon the initial position of the condyle. In the conservative approach, the goal of repositioning is a temporary one, with the aim of gradual resumption of the patient to the habitual condyle position, or to a concentric condyle position. This is achieved by the progressive adjustment of the repositioning appliance over several weeks or months. It is hypothesised that repositioning therapy restores the integrity of the disc shape and stability, while at the same time effecting an improved muscle coordination.[1]

Repositioning appliances actively direct jaw closure from habitual occlusion to a symmetrical or asymmetrical forward point in the horizontal plane (fig. 7 (a)–(b)). The magnitude of mandibular movement is usually from 1 to 2 mm, perhaps slightly more in those individuals with Angle Class II occlusions. The repositioning appliance is similar to the stabilisation appliance[19] with the exception that there are deeper fossas incorporating guiding planes that direct the mandible forward upon full closure (figs 7 (a)–(b)). It does not matter whether the appliance is fitted to the upper or lower arch: in the upper arch, the guiding planes contact the anterior teeth, and in the lower arch they contact the premolars and first molar.[20] In the opinion of the author, patient compliance is better with the mandibular design. Owing to its deep fossa design, the establishment of smooth articulation is incorporated only after a preliminary period of more or less vertical function during closure movements. The correctly adjusted appliance should provide stable contact on all posterior teeth. The appliance should be worn at all times, but especially during eating, when the disc–condyle complex is put under greatest functional demand.[21] Initially, a brief interval of muscular tension may accompany this treatment.

A considerable drawback to repositioning therapy is the potential for irreversible occlusal changes in the form of a gap between the posterior teeth. Surprisingly, many patients proceed with this type of therapy despite their awareness that orthodontics may be required to re-establish orderly posterior contact (fig. 8 (a)–(d)). Alternative tactics at this point entail selective occlusal adjustment, if feasible, or wearing the appliance at night, anticipating passive eruption during other times. Occasionally some patients return to their normal occlusal position without definitive care or complication.

Because repositioning therapy is somewhat unconventional, it is important to consider whether the same results might have been gained by traditional stabilisation appliance therapy. Unfortunately information about this comparison is sparse. Judging from clinical opinion, attempts to eliminate the clicking symptom by repositioning have been met with less than 50% success. However, Clark[18] found that 86% of patients who completed treatment found temporomandibular repositioning to be moderately to highly successful (50–100% improvement) at reducing the problems associated with TMJ clicking. Patients may show some improvement with a stabilisation appliance, but authors of two studies[17, 18] did not consider this a successful treatment for problems associated with clicking. These results support the point made by many clinicians that the criteria for successful repositioning therapy should not be based on the elimination of clicking in itself. The acceptable long-term results[22] of simple treatments for mandibular dysfunction involving clicking and locking suggest that the added difficulty in using repositioning techniques should be reserved for selected cases.

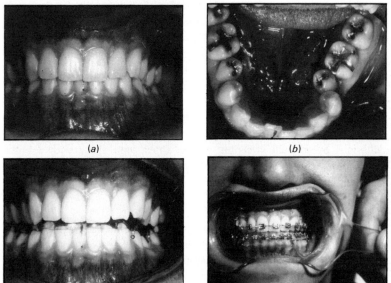

(a)

(b)

(c)

(d)

Fig. 8 Twenty-two-year-old male with troublesome clicking and incipient locking in the left TMJ. (*a*) Mandibular mid-line discrepancy towards the left side. (*b*) Occlusal view of the mandibular arch showing collapsed left posterior teeth. (*c*) Mandibular repositioning tests resulted in bringing the mandibular mid-lines into correct relationship. Note slight clockwise rotation of the mandible. (*d*) Eighteen months after beginning orthodontic treatment; note normalisation of the mid-lines.

Locking

Sudden onset of jaw restriction, known as locking, offers an opportunity to quickly re-establish range of motion and decrease pain. Manipulative reduction[3, 23] should be attempted when locking is suspected, but if its duration is determined to be more than one to two months, it is likely that other measures will need to be considered, as discussed below (fig. 9

(a)–(b)). The aim is to mobilise the TMJ in order to gain greater range of jaw motion (fig. 9(c)). If positive results are achieved, a repositioning appliance should be immediately fabricated and inserted that day, if possible (fig. 9(d)). Follow-up appointments for additional mobilisation should be performed in conjunction with a home exercise programme to maintain range of jaw motion. Although the results of this therapy cannot be said to achieve high success, those cases where results are obtained are gratifying to the patient, who otherwise might face a prolonged period of disabling restriction and discomfort. Often, patients with this therapy develop minor recurrent clicking which is either well tolerated or treated aggressively with longer term repositioning therapy.

Persistent locking leaves few options for management. If the patient can tolerate the restriction and accompanying functional pain, time is consonant with gradual resolution. About 50% of the pain associated with persistent locking can be ameliorated by the use of a stabilisation appliance used over variable periods of time. Recently, arthroscopy has been reported[24,25] to yield good results when employed on patients suffering from persistent locking. These reports describe the interruption of adhesions by manual sweeping of the upper joint space with a blunt probe,[24] and even by pumping solutions under pressure into the upper joint space, followed by manipulation.[25]

Arthroplasty

Surgical approaches to the management of TMJD embrace two techniques: disc repair and disc removal. The decision to do arthroplasty is dependent on the confirmed diagnosis of displacement of the articular disc and its role as a major source of the patient's pain and/or dysfunction.[26] It is estimated that no more than 5% of patients with TM disorders are candidates for arthroplasty. In North America, arthrography has played a large role in establishing the surgical diagnosis, and continues to be the procedure of

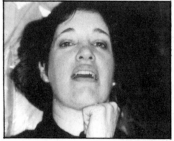

(a)   (b)

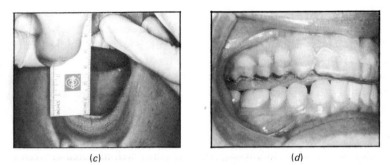

(c)   (d)

Fig. 9 Successful manipulation of locking in a 39-year-old woman complaining of soreness and restriction in the left TMJ. (*a*) Prop between ipsilateral molars provides for preliminary stretching of the TMJ capsule. (*b*) Mandible is manipulated downward, forward, and to the contralateral side. (*c*) Mouth opening was increased from 26 mm to 42 mm. (*d*) Temporary repositioning appliance was placed immediately using vacuum-pressed template and autopolymerising resin.

choice. TMJD patients with displacement of the articular disc without reduction (stage two and three) constitute a large share of those having TMJ surgery. This group has been shown to have more pain, more signs of dysfunction, and more hard tissue changes than those with disc displacement with reduction (stage one).[27] The surgical results are generally successful, even for the disc removal.[28] Most surgeons strongly recommend careful patient selection and integrated physical therapy in treatment.

Conclusion
Since the 1980s, there has been evidence that clicking and locking, previously thought to be part of the myofascial pain–dysfunction syndrome (MPD),[29] were actually due to observable TMJ changes. As a result, much more importance has been given to the differentiation of muscular disorders, TMJD, and synovitis. Of these three subgroups, TMJD is perhaps the most common. TMJD can be recognised by the predictable clusters of symptoms and signs which are best evaluated over time, and their recognition has suggested unique modes of treatment. Unlike the isolated model presented in this article, TMJD blends with masticatory muscle problems and tension headache complaints in the clinical setting, further complicating diagnosis. It has been stated that the decision to treat should not be made on identifying the existence of symptoms, but should rather depend upon their severity in consideration of patient motivation for immediate relief while at the same time keeping in mind the gradual tendency for TMJD to resolve over time.

Changes associated with TMJD affect centric relation and dental occlusion.[12] These factors should be taken into account when significant occlusal therapy is being performed. As a result of greater understanding of TMJD, alternative approaches to those traditionally employed have been suggested, including so-called mandibular repositioning. Therefore, increased attention to clinical and radiological assessment of TMJs is gaining importance in patient care.

References

1 Moffett B C, Westesson P-L, *Diagnosis of internal derangements of the temporomandibular joint Vol. 1: Double-contrast arthrography and clinical correlation.* 115 pp. Seattle: University of Washington Continuing Dental Education, 1984.

2 Solberg W K, Clark G T. *Temporomandibular joint problems: biological diagnosis and treatment.* 177 pp. Chicago: Quintessence, 1980.

3 Blankestijn J, Boering G. Posterior dislocation of the temporomandibular disc. *Int J Oral Surg* 1985; **14:** 437–443.

4 Ireland V E. The problem of the clicking jaw. *J Prosthet Dent* 1953; **3:** 200–212.

5 Farrar W B. Differentiation of temporomandibular joint dysfunction to simplify treatment. *J Prosthet Dent* 1972; **28:** 629–636.

6 Wilkes C H. Arthrography of the temporomandibular joint in patients with the TMJ pain–dysfunction syndrome. *Minn Med* 1978; **61:** 645–652.

7 Westesson P-L. Double-contrast arthrography of the temporomandibular joint. Introduction of an arthrographic technique for visualisation of the disc and articular surfaces. *J Oral Maxillofac Surg* 1983; **41:** 163–172.

8 Eriksson L, Westesson P-L, Rohlin M. Temporomandibular joint sounds correlated to function and morphology of the joint in patients with disk displacement. *Int J Oral Surg* 1985; **14:** 229–237.

9 Isberg-Holm A M, Westesson P-L. Movement of the disc and condyle in temporomandibular joints with clicking. An arthrographic and coneradiographic study on autopsy specimens. *Acta Odontol Scand* 1982; **40:** 153–166.

10 Rasmussen O C. Description of population and progress of symptoms in a longitudinal study of temporomandibular arthropathy. *Scand J Dent Res* 1981; **89:** 196–203.

11 McCarty W Jr. Diagnosis and treatment of internal derangements of the articular disc and mandibular condyle. *In* Solberg W K, Clark G T (eds) *Temporomandibular joint problems: biologic diagnosis and treatment.* pp 145–168. Chicago: Quintessence, 1980.

12 Isberg A, Widmalm S E, Ivarsson R. Clinical, radiographic and electromyographic study of patients with internal derangement of the temporomandibular joint. *Am J Orthod* 1985; **88:** 543–460.

13 Egermark-Eriksson I, Carlsson G E, Ingervall B. Prevalence of mandibular dysfunction and orofacial parafunction in 7-, 11-, and 15-year-old Swedish children. *Eur J Orthod* 1981; **3:** 163–172.

14 Solberg W K, Woo M S, Houston J B. Prevalence of mandibular dysfunction in young adults. *J Am Dent Assoc* 1979; **98:** 25–34.

15 Ricketts R M. Abnormal function of the temporomandibular joint. *Am J Orthod* 1955; **41:** 435–441.

16 Gerber A. Logik und mystik der kiefergelenkbeschwerden. *Schweiz Mschr Zahnheilk* 1964; **74:** 687–697.

17 Anderson G C, Schulte J K, Goodchild R J. Comparative study of two treatment methods for internal derangement of the temporomandibular joint. *J Prosthet Dent* 1985; **53:** 392–397.

18 Clark G T. Treatment of jaw clicking with temporomandibular repositioning: analysis of 25 cases. *J Craniomandib Pract* 1984; **2:** 263–270.

19 Solberg W K. Temporomandibular disorders: masticatory myalgia and its management. *Br Dent J* 1986; **160**: 351–356.

20 Clark G T. The temporomandibular joint repositioning appliance: a technique for construction, insertion and adjustment. *J Craniomandib Pract* 1986; **4**: 37–46.

21 Solberg W K. Temporomandibular disorders: functional and radiological considerations. *Br Dent J* 1986; **160**: 195–200.

22 Mejersjo C, Carlsson G E. Long term results of treatment for temporomandibular pain and dysfunction. *J Prosthet Dent* 1983; **49**: 809–815.

23 Solberg W K. Temporomandibular disorders: physical tests in diagnosis. *Br Dent J* 1986; **160**: 273–277.

24 Sanders B. Arthroscopic surgery of the temporomandibular joint. Treatment of internal derangement with persistent closed lock. *Oral Surg* 1986; (in press).

25 Murakami K-I, Matsuki M, Iizuka T, Ono T. Recapturing of persistent anterially displaced disc by mandibular manipulation after pumping and hydraulic pressure to the upper cavity of the temporomandibular joint. *J Craniomandib Prac* 1987; (in press).

26 Dolwick M F, Sanders B. *TMJ internal derangement and arthrosis*. 321pp. St Louis: C. V. Mosby, 1985.

27 Eriksson L, Westesson P-L. Clinical and radiological study of patient with anterior disk displacement of the temporomandibular joint. *Sws Dent J* 1983; **7**: 55–64.

28 Eriksson L, Westesson P-L. Long-term evaluation of meniscectomy of the temporomandibular joint. *J Oral Maxillofac Surg* 1985; **43**: 263–269.

29 Laskin D M. Etiology of the pain–dysfunction syndrome. *J Am Dent Assoc* 1969; **79**: 147–153.

8 Management of problems associated with inflammation, chronic hypomobility, and deformity

Temporomandibular disorders (TMD) consist of at least four major subgroups: muscular disorders, internal derangement, inflammatory disorders and conditions of hypomobility. Inflammatory disorders are capsular and synovial conditions which have arthralgia as their most prominent symptom. Less acknowledged are inflammations of the muscles and tendons that invite treatment in a manner analogous to synovitis. Although inflammatory pains are less common than myofascial complaints or internal derangement, their persistence and disabling effect on jaw function tend to push other complaints into the background and make their recognition by the practitioner a key to optimal patient management.

Loss of the condylar structure, whether associated with inflammation or non-inflammatory degenerative processes, may lead to complaints of bite dysfunction. The occlusal interferences are often mistaken as signs of inherent occlusal dysfunction, thus leading to attempts to correct what may be an ongoing problem of an unstable temporomandibular joint (TMJ).

Hypomobility disorders are problems not of pain, but of limited movement. Some hypomobility disorders, whether caused by the muscles or joints, follow in the footsteps of acute inflammation and signal the observer that fibrous changes are underway.

The purpose of this paper is to discuss the diagnosis and management of temporomandibular inflammation, deformity and hypomobility within the same context. The justification for this approach is that these are often closely allied conditions and that their management is best formulated by the practitioner having a perspective on rheumatological approaches, among others.

Temporomandibular inflammatory disorders

Inflammation may be localised or generalised, and these categories may be further differentiated into acute or chronic. Inflammation may be due to trauma, dysfunctional overload, osteoarthrosis, polyarthritis or infection. The detection of TMJ inflammation is reliably accomplished by palpation, by functional loading, and manipulation.[1] The use of radiographs and serology is diagnostically helpful for some types of synovitis, but is no substitute for a thorough clinical history and examination. Differential diagnosis includes potential infections as evidenced by fever, lymphadenopathy, swelling or malaise.[2]

Localised inflammation

Selected parts of the capsule or the disc attachments can be traumatised by functional overload or in association with faulty maxillomandibular relationships. The lateral (temporomandibular) ligament and the mediolateral and posterior disc attachments are the main sites involved. Posterior attachment inflammation sometimes becomes known in the course of routine dental procedures such as retruding the jaw in bite adjustment. Posterior TMJ tenderness may be confirmed by palpating via the ear canal. This step is important in order to help rule out joint pain referred from the sternocleidomastoid muscle, for example. Localised impingement is suspected if the pain is provoked by biting on a tongue blade on the contralateral side and if it is ameliorated by ipsilateral bitestick testing.[1] Lateral ligament inflammation may be confirmed by the finding of tenderness over the lateral aspect of the joint. Movements that stretch the lateral ligament will provoke the pain, such as wide open movements. These conditions vary in severity but do not usually approach the intensity of pain associated with acute synovitis.

Treatment should be directed at the cause, if known. For example, vigorous bruxism on the ipsilateral canine seems to produce inflammation in the lateral ligament. Localised inflammations often accompany internal derangement or muscular symptoms, in which case treatment of the most fundamental of these presentations is advisable. If posterior attachment pain is due to displacement of the disc, then measures should be taken to stabilise the disc.[3] If the inflammations occur secondary to overstretching of a joint capsule with fibrous contracture, direct treatment toward lessening the forces that bring tension on the joint. Bite appliances are successful in treating localised joint inflammation, when combined with applications of moist heat, gentle movement and rest. These localised therapies are usually sufficient to resolve the problem without the need for analgesics or anti-inflammatory drugs.

Synovitis

Synovitis (arthritis) occurs prominently in patients with active rheumatoid arthritis and secondarily through extension from other TMJ arthropathy.[4] Post-traumatic arthritis is usually expressed as a synovitis, in the presence or absence of hemarthrosis.[4] Synovitis is characterised by resting pain in the joint made worse by any movement. Almost any functional demand causes discomfort, as distinguished by localised inflammations whose symptoms are provoked only by specific jaw movements. The site of pain is well localised, causing the patient to use one finger to indicate the source of the symptoms.

The acute stage is described as a 'hot' joint because of the abruptness of onset and intensity of the symptoms. Swelling, if present, and pain cause abrupt functional restriction and secondary muscular splinting. Sudden bite discrepancy might be caused by associated oedema in the posterior attachment. Radiographic changes may be minimal, and should not be taken as a negative sign for TMJ pathology. Indeed, marked radiographic changes may be observed in the otherwise asymptomatic contralateral joint, indicating pre-existing latent TMJ changes. The prognosis often hinges upon the aetiology: a prior history of trauma, stress-related forceful clenching, or history of rheumatoid arthritis (RA). Synovitis may be due to an abrupt flare-up of a long-standing TMJ osteoarthrosis or as a sequela to the surgically treated TMJ. The diagnosis of these conditions would be supported by the history, radiographic and structural abnormalities, and in the case of RA, by serological tests.

Treatment of acute synovitis includes gentle icing of the affected area for 10-minute periods, rest, liquid diet, and mild analgesics. Centrally acting narcotic analgesics are generally ineffective in musculoskeletal pain of all types and are considered unwarranted for analgesia in patients with chronic rheumatic disease.[5] Ultrasound and other physiotherapy to the joint are an accepted option. As resolution of the acute stage commences, moist heat taken for 20-minute periods can be helpful in reducing inflammation and

Table I Old and newer non-steroidal analgesic anti-inflammatory drugs for management of inflammatory joint disease. (Excerpted from Nuki[5].)

Approved name	Proprietary name	Dose
Soluble aspirin	Solprin	600 mg × 6 daily
Diflunisal	Dolobid	500 mg × 2 daily
Ibuprofen	Brufen	400–600 mg × 4 daily
Sulindac	Clinoril	200 mg × 2 daily
Piroxicam	Feldene	20 mg daily

associated muscular effects. The course of symptoms depends upon the aetiology, but could be as short as a few days if, for example, the cause were a single stressful event involving forceful clenching (figs 1 (*a*)–(*c*)). If the above procedures are considered insufficient to ameliorate the symptoms of severe synovitis, non-steroidal analgesic anti-inflammatory drugs (NSAIDs) are the most commonly accepted therapy. Selected NSAIDs and their doses are listed in Table I. All of these agents have analgesic, anti-inflammatory, and antipyretic activity.[5] Among other effects, NSAIDs inhibit the synthesis of prostaglandins and desensitise blood vessels to the permeability effects of other mediators of inflammation. The same effects are responsible for their propensity to cause gastrointestinal irritation.[5]

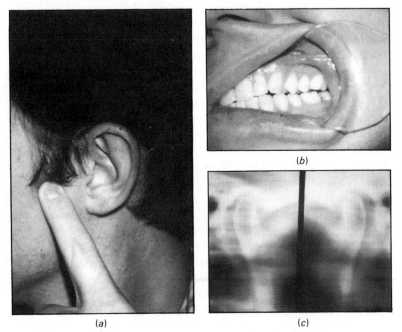

(*a*)   (*c*)

Fig. 1 Young man complaining of TM disorder following a stressful day: (*a*) swelling over the left TMJ; (*b*) disruption of the bite (*c*) protruded relationship of the mandibular condyle consistent with effusion and oedema in the joint. Presumptive aetiology is forceful clenching during stress. Resolution was uneventful within 10 days.

These drugs are effective analgesics, and if analgesia is the chief goal, the shorter-acting ones (aspirin, ibuprofen) should be prescribed 'on demand'. If anti-inflammatory levels are desired, then time-contingent doses at anti-inflammatory levels are necessary. Because the response is significantly variable between individuals, it is recommended to try at least one other NSAID if the first trial fails.[5]

Injections of corticosteroids into the superior TMJ space are effective in suppressing synovitis but they are not to be employed on a regular basis (fig. 2).[6,7] Nevertheless, intra-articular injections of corticosteroids in patients with synovitis have been controversial owing to the concern over destruction of articular tissue following injection of these agents.[8,9]

Kopp and Wenneberg[10] compared the efficacy of occlusal therapy and corticosteroid injections on patients with tenderness and pain in the TMJs. Both treatments reduced the signs and symptoms, but the reduction was significantly greater among those who received joint injections. These findings are particularly significant considering that the injection group had previously failed to respond to occlusal therapy. It seemed that intra-articular injections had the best effect on those patients free of radiographic changes and having a full set of natural teeth.

Systemic administration of corticosteroids may be justified in some cases of arthritis, but most rheumatologists are reluctant to use them in cases of uncomplicated synovitis.[7] However, intra-articular injections of corticosteroids are administered with considerable success in RA. This is usually carried out for one or two troublesome joints that are resistant to a general programme. Thus, dental consultants may receive requests to make injections from rheumatologists unfamiliar with the technique of injecting the TMJ. If the first injection is not effective, a second may be given after

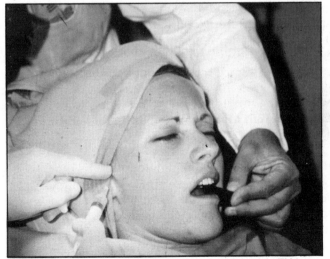

Fig. 2 Intra-articular injection of the superior joint space of the right TMJ.

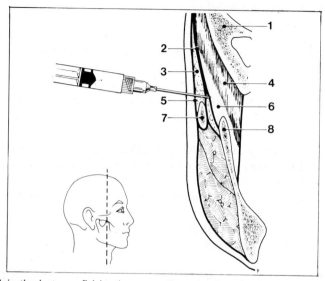

Fig. 3 Injection just superficial to the temporalis tendon: (1) cranium; (2) deep temporalis fascia; (3) fat pad; (4) temporalis muscle; (5) superficial temporalis fascia; (6) temporalis tendon; (7) zygoma; (8) coronoid process. Dotted line denotes plane of view.

a period of two weeks. If the second one fails, other attempts are likely to be unsuccessful.[7]

In summary, synovitis is recognised by focal joint pain and restriction of continuous aching character that is substantiated by palpation of the joint. In the presence of an acute synovitis, the patient will point unequivocally to that joint. The resolution of acute synovitis can be uneventful, but when persistent, anti-inflammatory medications in addition to physiotherapy and home care are indicated. Those likely to respond to intra-articular injections are individuals diagnosed with synovitis but free of TMJ radiographic changes those with a localised flare-up of RA.[8]

Tendinitis

Although myotendinopathy is an accepted clinical differentiation in the shoulder,[11] it has rarely been discussed in the context of temporomandibular disorders.[12] The temporalis tendon and its accompanying sheath are potentially reactive to excessive forces. These forces, whether due to macro- or microtrauma, result in chronic inflammation with characteristic functional pain and stiffness. Accordingly, treatment strategies include anti-inflammatory drugs and other measures that are appropriate for the treatment of inflammations, eg synovitis.

The temporalis tendon is mostly superficial to the muscle, and when palpated it has almost a bony character. It may be palpated at a site about 25 mm posterior to the orbital rim, just above the zygomatic arch (fig. 3). The lower part of the tendon may be approached via the buccal cavity, just above and medial to coronoid process. The diagnosis of tendinitis is made by the identification of discrete tenderness at the tendon site, and by the provocation of pain when applying resistance against the actively contracting jaw closers.[1] Clinically, tendinitis is manifested by resting pain over the tendon site and unilateral headache which is aggravated by vigorous chewing. Differentiation of tendon pain from muscle pain is dependent upon the site of tenderness. By comparision, the anterior portion of the temporalis muscle is well above and/or deep to the tendon site. Limitation of jaw motion is not significant, unless it is part of a larger problem such as RA or TMJ derangement.

Pain at the tendon site tends to resolve with methods already mentioned[13] to treat masticatory muscle disorders. However, specific treatment of tendinitis is appealing when it is desirable to give the patient demonstrable relief, for example, prior to bite appliance therapy. Alternatively, if tendon pain persists after conservative approaches fail to bring results, direct intervention should be considered. Injection of 1 ml 1% lignocaine directly superficial to the tendon is suggested as a diagnostic trial (fig. 3). Within 5 minutes after the injection, if the pain and/or restriction are significantly abated, a follow-up injection of 0·5 ml of betamethasone 6 mg per ml (Celestone Soluspan) is given at the same site (fig. 3). A perceptible resistance can be detected when at the correct depth, provided the needle is of sufficient width. Moderate tenderness and restriction may follow for two days before therapeutic benefit is seen. Injections may be repeated once or twice at 5-day intervals. Additional benefit is gained by supportive physical therapy in the form of heat and gentle movement. Patients with tendinitis should continue on an ultra-soft or liquid diet until symptoms diminish. Excessive function during the period of symptomatic relief will aggravate recovery or bring on renewed symptoms.

In summary, evidence to support corticosteroid therapy in tender spots over tendons in the masticatory region is anecdotal and unsubstantiated by clinically controlled trials, and its effect may be only temporary if forces that brought about the condition are not controlled. In six recent clinical cases where the author has employed this modality, four of the six had clear-cut benefit with subjects reporting from 50 to 100% improvement over the short term. Those using this technique should be familiar with the properties of the corticosteroids which are well recorded and will not be discussed here.

Chronic inflammation associated with osteoarthrosis

Osteoarthrosis (OA) is a common degenerative chronic condition that increases with age, and there is evidence that the condition is more severe in women than in men.[14] Articular tissue and subchrondral bone are the sites of major abnormalities in the osteoarthrotic process.[6] For this reason, OA is most often asymptomatic, but when symptoms develop, they are usually localised, obscure in onset, and unassociated with systemic manifestations.[15]

Synovitis is often seen as a clinical complication of OA, but the inflammatory changes are usually mild and secondary. NSAIDs are generally less effective than in rheumatoid arthritis.[5] Stabilisation appliances[13] are useful, and have the advantage of directing therapy against a potential aetiological factor in OA, namely repetitive impulse loading.[16] This view is supported by the evidence that molar tooth loss is an aetiological factor in the development of crepitation and probably TMJ–OA.[17,18] Therefore, for the TMJ–OA patient having occlusal and mandibular instability, the appropriate therapy is the stabilisation bite appliance. The interval between appliance delivery and resolution of symptoms is usually longer than for muscular disorders. Many of these patients subsequently enter a second phase of occlusal therapy involving orthodontics and prosthodontics (figs 4 (a)–(f)). Others wear a bite appliance at night indefinitely in order to maintain their symptom-free status (figs5 (a)–(b)).

Education and reassurance about the disease, avoidance of excessive joint strain, and physical therapy aimed at relieving pain and encouraging adequate range of motion are good approaches to overall management of symptomatic OA. Heat is applied in the form of hot packs, ultrasound, or diathermy.[6] Muscular exercises should be approached with caution and are best utilised gradually without putting the joint through extreme ranges of motion. Surgery to the TMJ, including meniscectomy,[19] is a viable alternative in severe cases where chronic pain and limited function continue to create meaningful disability. If there is doubt whether the primary source of the pain is in the TMJ, the auriculotemporal nerve block[20] can be employed (fig. 6).

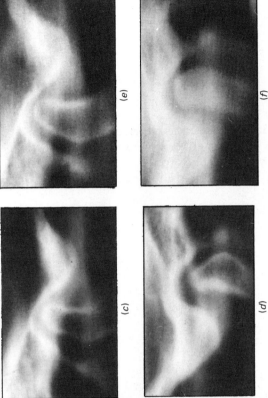

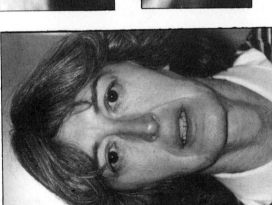

Fig. 4 (*a*) Fifty three-year-old patient with moderate-to-severe synovitis associated with osteoarthrosis. (*b*) Unstable occlusion rectified by the fitting of a bite appliance. (*c*) Right and (*d*) left TMJ tomograms at first visit. (*e*) Right and (*f*) left TMJ tomograms after 4 months' bite appliance therapy followed by 3 years full-banded orthodontic treatment. Note apparent shape changes in the condyles of both joints after treatment. Tomograms shown here were taken using a cephalostat and identical depth of cut on the same x-ray unit.

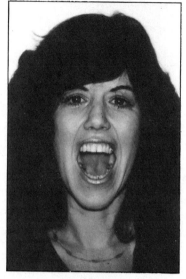

(a)

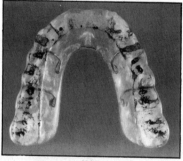

(b)

Fig. 5 (a) Thirty-five-year-old patient originally seen with a severe synovitis but unsuccessfully treated with multiple injections of corticosteroid. She has remained symptom-free only if she continues to wear her (b) maxillary bite appliance, pictured here after 10 years' use. Markings show areas of tooth contact movement. Note full range of jaw motion after treatment.

Disorders associated with bite dysfunction and deformity

Rheumatoid arthritis is the most common inflammatory polyarthritis affecting humans,[7] and in the dental setting, bite dysfunction is a common complaint. Rheumatoid arthritis is three times more common in women than in men, and the mean age of onset is about 40 years in both sexes.[21]

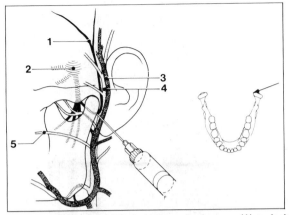

Fig. 6 Anaesthetic blockade of the left auriculotemporal nerve: (1) auriculotemporal nerve; (2) semilunar ganglion, trigeminal nerve; (3) superficial temporalis vein; (4) superficial temporalis artery; (5) transverse facial artery. The needle is placed just anteromedially to the condylar neck. Anterior direction, to the left. Arrow depicts needle orientation in the horizontal plane.

Temporomandibular pain is not usually a prominent symptom, and RA usually does not cause demonstrable jaw limitation.[22] For a review of RA in the TMJs, see other sources.[21,23]

The treatment of TMJ pain in RA is dealt with mostly in the context of an overall medical programme supplemented by intra-articular injections of corticosteroid (discussed above). Rarely is a bite appliance a critical modality for controlling the joint pain associated with RA. On the other hand, dental procedures are frequently needed to deal with masticatory

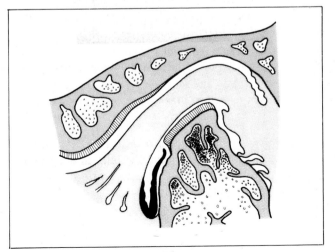

(a)

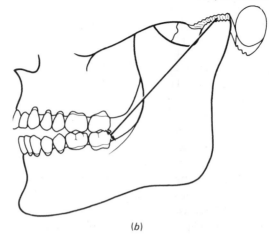

(b)

Fig. 7 (a) Drawing of TMJ with rheumatoid arthritis, with pannus eroding condyle from the anterior and posterior. Unaffected normal disc and central superior portion of the condyle. (b) Drawing of mandibular position resulting from condylar erosion in rheumatoid arthritis. Note fibrous ankylosis and shortened condyle. Closure on the decreased radius results in occlusal contact on the distal of the second molars producing a retruded, anterior open bite. (From Manan P E. The tempormandibular joint in function and dysfunction. *In* Solberg W K, Clark G T(eds) *Temporomandibular joint problems: biologic diagnosis and treatment.* pp 40-41. Chicago: Quintessence, 1980.)

disability and open bite (figs 7 (a)–(b)). Bite appliances worn during meal times often give ongoing benefit to RA sufferers with associated bite complaints. These appliances 'fill the gap' and thereby decrease the secondary muscle pain while improving the trituration of food. Use of these appliances during sleep achieves additional stabilisation, should there be nocturnal bruxism.

Dibbets *et al.*[24] have described a condition in children which they have termed arthrosis deformans juvenilis (ADJ). They have defined ADJ as consisting of clicking or pain plus radiographic findings of deformation of the mandibular condyles. Morphometric analyses on the ADJ group whose mean age was twelve years and six months indicated 'a shorter corpus dominated in a smaller mandible' in the group with deviant contour of one of the condyles.[24] These authors considered the dysfunctional findings to be indicators of specific growth patterns. Treatment involves establishing the most appropriate maxillomandibular development possible with less specialised management of the TMJ changes. The early development of ADJ might explain why young adults may later complain of symptoms of classic, but premature osteoarthritis.

Osteorthrosis tends to produce insidious changes in the occlusion from proliferative and regressive remodelling (figs 8 (*a*)–(*d*)). Some growth disorders such as condylar hyperplasia and osteochondroma work to move the mandible forward and to the contralateral side. Various other abnormalities of growth such as condylar hypoplasia, neoplasia and dual bite are often accompanied by latent mandibular dysfunction or functional pain.

These findings are treated after radiographically evaluating the nature of the functional problem. Progressive occlusal adjustment of the teeth (coronoplasty) may be sufficient to cope with the details of occlusal fit and function. The patient should be aware that further disease progression may undo what gains have been made by this procedure.

Occasionally the complaint is one of sudden posterior bite discrepancy in the older patient, This usually occurs secondary to jamming of the partially destroyed articular disc. Radiographic evaluation invariably reveals gross changes in the TMJs. If the discrepancy persists, prosthetic treatment to rectify the minor bite discrepancy is usually effective.

Chronic hypomobility
Painless restriction of mouth opening can be associated with mechanical contracture of the TMJ capsule and masticatory muscles, with adhesions between the articular disc and joint surface, and with bony ankylosis. Individuals having these problems may have a long history of temporomandibular disorders or systemic disease such as scleroderma. The main process underlying these problems is fibrous deposition in the muscle and joint tissues.

The findings are obvious. Diminished freeway space, limited opening accompanied by a hard 'end-feel', stiffness to the tissues, and palpably abnormal condylar function. Because the restriction is physical rather than physiological, treatment measures that work in other TM disorder subgroups result in equivocal success for chronic hypomobility disorders. For example, anticipated restoration of range of motion with a bite appliance is unrealistic.

Other causes of hypomobility are less obscure, such as bony obstruction (fig. 9), tumours, or gross trauma. Their proper course of treatment is also more evident. Clinical and radiological efforts should be made to find the cause of the hypomobility and to inform the patient of the options, which may include therapeutic arthroscopy, arthroplasty, myotomy or no specific treatment.

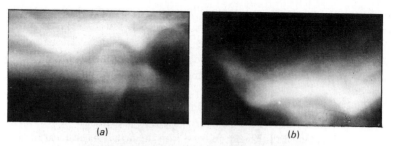

(a)   (b)

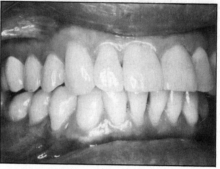

(c)

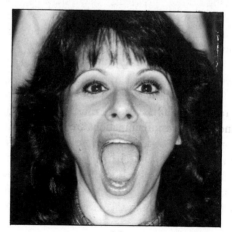

(d)

Fig. 8 Tomograph of (*a*) left TMJ at first visit of a 32-year-old patient experiencing mild arthralgia and myalgia. (*b*) Tomograph of the same joint taken three years later revealing marked osteoarthosis. (*c*) Complaints of bite discomfort, but no pain, were expressed at follow-up. (*d*) Despite the severe TMJ changes, range of opening remained normal.

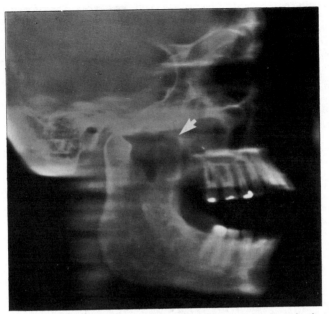

Fig. 9 Fifty-year-old woman with restricted opening secondary to bony impingement caused by elongation of the coronoid process. There were concomitant radiographic findings of OA in both TMJs. This case was treated surgically to remove the overdeveloped bony process.

Conclusion

Because of their tenacious persistence, inflammatory disorders and their late sequelae must be reckoned with among the subgroups making up TM disorders. The recognition of TMJ inflammation is rather easily identified, but muscular and tendinous inflammations are less obvious. As was the case for myalgia[13] and TMJ internal derangement[3] familiarity with the characteristics of inflammatory disorders offers specific treatment options that insure greater predictability in patient outcome. Greater understanding of the therapeutic limitations of most hypomobility disorders brings forth more enlightened patient management.

Acknowledgements

Grateful appreciation is extended to Irene Petrivicius of UCLA Dental Illustration and to Patricia Smiley for her aid in preparing the manuscripts.

References

1 Solberg W K. Temporomandibular disorders: physical tests in diagnosis. *Br Dent J* 1986; **160**: 273–277.

2 Carlsson G E, Kopp S, Oberg T. Arthritis and allied diseases of the temporomandibular joint. *In* Zarb G A, Carlsson G E (eds) *Temporomandibular joint function and dysfunction.* pp 269–320. Copenhagen: Munksgaard, 1979.

3 Solberg W K. Temporomandibular disorders: management of internal derangement. *Br Dent J* 1986; **160**: 379–385.

4 Bell W E. *Temporomandibular disorders: classification, diagnosis, management.* 2nd ed, pp 173–214. London: Yearbook Publishers, 1986.

5 Nuki G. Non-steroidal analgesic and anti-inflammatory agents. *Br Med J* 1983; **287**: 39–43.

6 Moskowitz R W. Management of osteoarthritis. *Bull Rheum Dis* 1981 series; **31**: 31–35.

7 Hunder G G, Bunch T W. Treatment of rheumatoid arthritis. *Bull Rheum Dis* 1982 series; **32**: 1–10.

8 Wenneberg B, Kopp S. Short term effect of intra-articular injections of a corticosteroid on the temporomandibular joint pain and dysfunction. *Swed Dent J* 1978; **2**: 189–196.

9 Toller P A. Use and misuse of intra-articular corticosteroids in treatment of temporomandibular joint pain. *Proc R Soc Med* 1977; **70**: 461–463.

10 Kopp S, Wenneberg B. Effects of occlusal treatment and intra-articular injections of temporomandibular joint pain and dysfunction. *Acta Odontol Scand* 1981; **39**: 87–96.

11 Calabro J J, Londino A V Jr, Eyvazzadeh C. Sustained-release indomethacin in the management of the acute painful shoulder from bursitis and/or tendinitis. *Am J Med* 1985; **74**: 32–38.

12 Friedman M H. Tenomyositis of the masseter muscle: report of cases. *J Am Dent Assoc* 1985; **110**: 201–202.

13 Solberg W K. Temporomandibular disorders: masticatory myalgia and its management. *Br Dent J* 1986; **160**: 351–356.

14 Davis M A. Sex differences in reporting osteoarthritic symptoms: a sociomedical approach. *J Health Soc Behav* 1981; **22**: 298–310.

15 Kopp S. Subjective symptoms in temporomandibular joint osteoarthrosis. *Acta Odont Scand* 1977; **35**: 207–215.

16 Radin E L. Mechanical aspects of osteoarthrosis. *Bull Rheum Dis* 1975–76 series; **26**: 862–865.

17 Kopp S. Clinical findings in temporomandibular joint osteoarthrosis. *Scand J Dent Res* 1977; **85**: 434–443.

18 Öberg T, Carlsson G E, Fajers C-M. The temporomandibular joint. A morphologic study on a human autopsy material. *Acta Odontol Scand* 1971; **29**: 349–384.

19 Eriksson L, Westersson P-L. Long-term evaluation of meniscectomy of the temporomandibular joint. *J Oral Maxillofac Surg* 1985; **43**: 263–269.

20 Donlon W C, Truta M P, Eversole L R. A modified auriculotemporal nerve block for regional anesthesia of the temporomandibular joint. *J Maxillofac Surg* 1984; **42**: 544–555.

21 Ogus H. Rheumatoid arthritis of the temporomandibular joint. *Br J Oral Surg* 1975; **12**: 275–284.

22 Larheim T A, Floystrand T. Temporomandibular joint abnormalities and bite force in a group of adults with rheumatoid arthritis. *J Oral Rehab* 1985; **12**: 477–482.

23 Franks A S T. Temporomandibular joint in adult rheumatoid arthritis. A comparative evaluation of 100 cases. *Ann Rheum Dis* 1969; **28**: 139–145.

24 Dibbets J M H, Van Der Weele L T, Uildriks A K J. Symptoms of TMJ dysfunction: Indicators of growth patterns? *J Pedodontics* 1985; **9**: 265–284.